AF790359

Contemporary Topics in Patient Safety - Volume 3

Edited by Philip N. Salen
and Stanislaw P. Stawicki

Published in London, United Kingdom

Contemporary Topics in Patient Safety - Volume 3
http://dx.doi.org/10.5772/intechopen.1001685
Edited by Philip N. Salen and Stanislaw P. Stawicki

Contributors
Adel Omar Bataweel, Alaa Mahmoud Ismail, Amin Ataie, An Goldbauer, Chukwuma Richard Uzoka, Denice Curtis, Ebrahim Sarwi Asiri, Grace M. Arteaga, Hesham Ahmed Eid, Jameelah Mohammed Yaqoob, James Fallah, Khaled M. Kasasbeh, LaRissa Adams, Milad Esmaeilzadeh Farmad, Mohamed Fathy Shaban, Mohammed M. Albaadani, Nasr Ali Mohammed, Nazri Nordin, Opal Davidson, Pablo Moreno Franco, Parisa Saberi-Hasanabadi, Philip N. Salen, Ramin Ataee, Romana Jelínková, Samir Mohammed Bawazir, Sandy C. Booth, Siham Mohammed Saleh, Stanislaw P. Stawicki, Yasser Sami Amer

© The Editor(s) and the Author(s) 2024

The rights of the editor(s) and the author(s) have been asserted in accordance with the Copyright, Designs and Patents Act 1988. All rights to the book as a whole are reserved by INTECHOPEN LIMITED. The book as a whole (compilation) cannot be reproduced, distributed or used for commercial or non-commercial purposes without INTECHOPEN LIMITED's written permission. Enquiries concerning the use of the book should be directed to INTECHOPEN LIMITED rights and permissions department (permissions@intechopen.com).

Violations are liable to prosecution under the governing Copyright Law.

CC BY

Individual chapters of this publication are distributed under the terms of the Creative Commons Attribution 3.0 Unported License which permits commercial use, distribution and reproduction of the individual chapters, provided the original author(s) and source publication are appropriately acknowledged. If so indicated, certain images may not be included under the Creative Commons license. In such cases users will need to obtain permission from the license holder to reproduce the material. More details and guidelines concerning content reuse and adaptation can be found at http://www.intechopen.com/copyright-policy.html.

Notice

Statements and opinions expressed in the chapters are these of the individual contributors and not necessarily those of the editors or publisher. No responsibility is accepted for the accuracy of information contained in the published chapters. The publisher assumes no responsibility for any damage or injury to persons or property arising out of the use of any materials, instructions, methods or ideas contained in the book.

First published in London, United Kingdom, 2024 by IntechOpen
IntechOpen is the global imprint of INTECHOPEN LIMITED, registered in England and Wales, registration number: 11086078, 167-169 Great Portland Street, London, W1W 5PF, United Kingdom

British Library Cataloguing-in-Publication Data
A catalogue record for this book is available from the British Library

Additional hard and PDF copies can be obtained from orders@intechopen.com

Contemporary Topics in Patient Safety - Volume 3
Edited by Philip N. Salen and Stanislaw P. Stawicki
p. cm.
Print ISBN 978-0-85466-716-1
Online ISBN 978-0-85466-715-4
eBook (PDF) ISBN 978-0-85466-717-8

We are IntechOpen, the world's leading publisher of Open Access books

Built by scientists, for scientists

7,200+
Open access books available

190,000+
International authors and editors

205M+
Downloads

156
Countries delivered to

Our authors are among the
Top 1%
most cited scientists

12.2%
Contributors from top 500 universities

WEB OF SCIENCE™

Selection of our books indexed in the Book Citation Index in Web of Science™ Core Collection (BKCI)

Interested in publishing with us?
Contact book.department@intechopen.com

Numbers displayed above are based on latest data collected.
For more information visit www.intechopen.com

For EU product safety concerns:
IN TECH d.o.o., Prolaz Marije Krucifikse Kozulić 3, 51000 Rijeka, Croatia,
info@intechopen.com or visit our website at intechopen.com.

Meet the editors

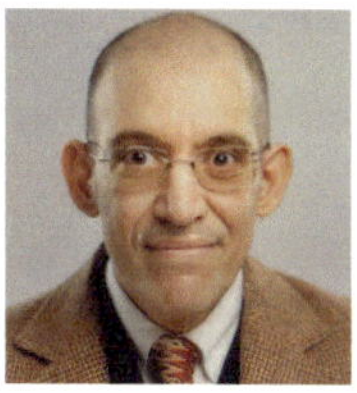

Dr. Phillip Salen is an Emergency Medicine Attending and Core Academic Faculty at the St. Luke's University Hospital Emergency Medicine Residency, PA. He is the Director of Research for the St. Luke's EM Residency and an adjunct clinical associate professor at the Lewis Katz School of Medicine, Temple University, Department of Emergency Medicine, PA. A specialist in emergency medicine, he has co-authored more than 110 scholarly works including journal manuscripts, book chapters, electronic book chapters, abstracts, and photo publications. Dr. Salen is a member of multiple editorial and review boards. His areas of expertise include emergency medicine ultrasound, medical education, patient safety, gastroenteritis, feeding tube complications, radiation safety, and improving emergency medicine clinician communication and wellness.

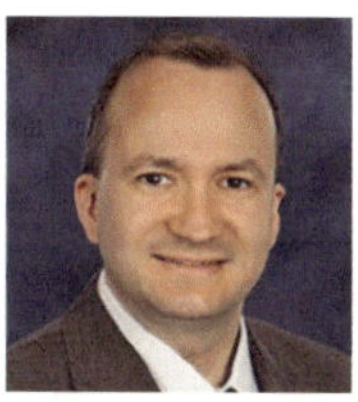

Dr. Stanislaw P. Stawicki is Professor of Surgery and Chair of the Department of Research and Innovation, St. Luke's University Health Network, PA. A specialist in trauma, general surgery, and surgical critical care, he has co-authored more than 670 scholarly works, including more than 25 books. In addition to national and international medical leadership roles, Dr. Stawicki is a member of numerous editorial boards and grant evaluation/review bodies. His areas of expertise include medical innovation, blockchain technology, medical education, patient safety, academic leadership, mentorship, trauma/critical care, and sonography.

Contents

Preface

Patient safety continues to be one of the most important topics in health care today. Despite several decades of progress, much collective work remains to be done before health systems worldwide reach the ultimate goal of "zero harm". The incidence and impact of unintentional iatrogenic harm is difficult to quantify, with an infinite combination of "moving parts" and their mutual interactions making the very process of "tracking progress" exceedingly difficult. That said, some health systems may be closer than others to that ultimate "zero harm" goal, yet none of the health systems are close to definitively completing this important mission.

As the global trek toward improved patient safety continues, the focus remains squarely on value-based care delivery, including better outcomes, improved quality, and enhanced safety. In addition, given increasingly constrained healthcare resources worldwide, a parallel focus on cost containment results in an environment that inherently competes with some patient safety goals (specifically affecting the ultimate amount of resources available to address existing critical patient safety shortcomings). This, in turn, mandates ongoing efforts to better understand and optimize all aspects of healthcare operations across all functional levels, from individual providers to clinics and hospitals, to administrative support, and ultimately, health systems from regional to global dimensions.

It is well established that healthcare-associated adverse events, or broadly defined "iatrogenic harm", play a significant role by affecting both clinical outcomes and systemic costs associated with care delivery. As individual patients journey across their personal healthcare path, the identification of various actual and potential safety events can be challenging, especially when taking the "real-time" or prospective approach. In general, patient safety events can be viewed as undesirable consequences to a healthcare process or procedure that is performed or implemented during a patient's healthcare encounter, no matter how "routine" in character. When stratifying patient safety events, one must recognize the critical importance of identifying and addressing the so-called "near misses" or "close calls", which represent circumstances where an adverse event did not occur or did not cause actual harm, but the potential for the same existed all along. Proceeding along the continuum of risk, typical categories of adverse events may include medication errors, catheter-related infections, healthcare-associated falls, wrong-site surgery, and communication or handoff breakdowns. Moreover, harm often occurs because of failures to act, failures to recognize/rescue, competency/knowledge/education gaps, inadequate skills, poor or impaired judgment, delays in care secondary to process or system (or staffing) challenges, as well as limited access to health care due to constrained resources and/or overwhelmed systemic capacity.

The impact of patient safety events is of course greatest and most immediate on the affected patients and their families. Associated impacts on the institution and the overall healthcare system are also profound, ranging from loss of trust to significantly greater costs of care delivery. In this context, we must factor in specific considerations, such as lost productivity, lower quality of life, greater need for testing and/or subsequent care, prolonged hospitalizations, and the impact on resources available to other patients. The latter is often "felt" in the form of environments that under-deliver due to limits on the ability to provide much needed care to a specific population or region.

It is important to note that breakdowns in patient safety can also have substantial effects on the healthcare team, with an especially high impact on bedside personnel, including nurses, allied health professionals, and physicians. Provider burnout continues to be a major concern across our healthcare settings, and although burnout can be attributed to a variety of factors, the personal and professional accountability (or sense of "failure") can result in difficult-to-alleviate emotional toll, especially on those directly involved in caring for patients. In this context, providers may experience feelings of inadequacy, powerlessness, or hopelessness when directly involved in patient safety breakdowns. This, in turn, can reflect a continuum of engagement, support, and/or enthusiasm, especially when the delivery of high-quality care requires the presence of a high-functioning, fully engaged, multidisciplinary team. To address some of the issues connecting patient safety lapses and burnout, we must emphasize the importance of strong, competent leadership, high-performance institutional culture, dedication to employee wellness, and team empowerment. A substantial amount of individual and team satisfaction can be derived from objective progress and improvements in patient safety, which can be considered as a "positive spiral" (in contrast to the "negative spiral" associated with patient safety events and burnout). This, in turn, can contribute significantly to a personally and professionally gratifying and healthy organizational environment. In a way, this concept exemplifies the adage, "a rising tide lifts all boats" when positive and constructive team behaviors lead to more positivity and the general feeling of collective accomplishment.

As healthcare institutions and teams continue on the patient safety trek, critical elements of organizational culture emerge as primary drivers of progress. This culture of safety represents an ongoing paradigm shift, with increasing emphasis on non-punitive exploration and analysis of patient safety events, focusing on opportunities to understand "how and why" patient safety issues evolve and develop. After all, system-wide improvements can only come when there is a broader understanding of why adverse events occur and what mechanisms are in place to prevent or mitigate them under the umbrella of assumption of innocence, goodwill, and fully acknowledging that no one is perfect. As our collective knowledge of patient safety and related topics grows, it becomes evident that initiatives focused on improving patient safety may have certain unintended consequences and may even lead to secondary downstream harm. Consequently, we need to recognize that any initiative to improve patient care by reducing risk and the potential for harm also requires continued vigilance, not only to ensure the desired goals are met but also to minimize any unintended consequences.

Philip N. Salen
Department of Emergency Medicine,
St. Luke's University Health Network,
Bethlehem, Pennsylvania, USA

Stanislaw P. Stawicki
Department of Research and Innovation,
St. Luke's University Health Network,
Bethlehem, Pennsylvania, USA

Chapter 1

Introductory Chapter: Enhancing Physician Wellness to Prevent Burnout Promotes Clinician and Patient Safety

Philip N. Salen and Stanislaw P. Stawicki

Ἰατρέ, θεράπευσον σεαυτόν (Physician heal thyself) Ancient Greek Proverb.

1. Introduction and objectives

Patient safety is central to modern healthcare delivery systems, with ever increasing focus on delivering the best possible, safest care, at cost levels that are both reasonable and sustainable [1]. In this third installment of Contemporary Issues in Patient Safety, we explore a host of interconnected topics that directly and indirectly affect the value- and safety-driven, patient-centric dynamic of today. Among the various topics explored in this book, provider burnout as a contributor to medical and surgical error deserves a much closer examination. The Editors would like to devote this Introductory Chapter to burnout, its insidious nature, as well as the need for recognition and prompt management.

2. Focus on provider burnout

Physician burnout has a major impact on patient safety, patient satisfaction, and healthcare outcomes. Physician burnout also has major implications for physician job satisfaction, longevity, and wellbeing. Data and information for this exploratory review was obtained via literature search that included PubMed, Medline, and Google Scholar. Fatigue, especially when working in intense clinical environments, prolonged shifts, and overnight shifts plays a major role in inducing burnout with resultant increases in medical errors, worse patient outcomes, and patient dissatisfaction with healthcare providers. Multiple strategies have been implemented to prevent and treat burnout including limiting work hours, incorporating sleep and exercise into shift-work, and engaging physician providers in administrative decision making.

Health professionals including physicians have reported high levels of emotional and physical burnout induced by a combination of factors including fatigue from extreme work hours, excessive overnight shift work, increasing amounts of administrative work, pandemic induced stress, and exposure to workplace violence [2].

IntechOpen

Physician burnout affects healthcare delivery by directly and indirectly impacting patient safety, patient outcomes, patient experience, and our overall ability to deliver effective and safe care throughout hospital networks. Burnout syndrome results from extreme professional demands, depersonalization in the work environment, excessive fatigue, and psychiatric depression, all of which combine to impair work performance and result in dissatisfaction in both personal and professional spheres [3–5]. Physician burnout results in a loss of sense of mission, diminished self-esteem, and progressive lack of enthusiasm, affecting one's ability to provide their best effort for patients [6].

Physician burnout commonly manifests as emotional lassitude, loss of empathy, depression, and feelings of lack of personal accomplishment [7, 8]. It tends to be a progressive and insidious process, often difficult to detect in its earlier and intermediate phases, and quite frequently does not manifest overtly until it is quite advanced [9, 10]. Clinician burnout impacts physicians' professionalism and effective communication with other providers [8]. Burnout does not appear to be related to number of years worked; medical students, physicians in training, and experienced attending physicians alike note emotional burnout, with emergency physicians reporting the highest levels among all specialties of up to 70% of practitioners [3, 9, 11]. Burnout impairs hampers compassionate communications with patients, lowers patient satisfaction, increases door-to-doctor waiting periods resulting in decreased number of patients seen per hour in the emergency department and other outpatient settings, and increases the odds of job dissatisfaction [3, 7, 12]. All these factors related to burnout impair work productivity and efficiency, increases the likelihood of safety accidents, exacerbates personal relationship difficulties of clinicians, increases readmission rates, and jeopardizes the overall safety and quality of health care provided [12–14]. In the current book, significant focus is placed on the phenomenon of physician burnout, various associated risk factors, as well as an in-depth discussion on the impact of physician burnout on patient safety and outcomes. Finally, we discuss different options for resolving and preventing burnout.

Many elements contribute to physician burnout including work induced anxiety, shift duration, excessive work hours especially hours worked overnight and during holidays, patient illness severity, number of patients cared for, excessive administrative responsibilities, frustration about the inability to address patients' needs, and inadequate clinical and emotional support in the workplace (See **Figure 1**) [5, 6]. Research has demonstrated the correlation of exhaustion and depression to independently and in combination provoke the likelihood that physicians in training will perceive that they have committed medical errors [15]. Public health crises such as the Covid epidemic from 2020 to 2022 place stress on the clinical work force, including physicians and nurses. Nearly 20% of 9300 surveyed physicians and 40% of surveyed nurses in a Coping with COVID questionnaire noted that they had considered retirement from medical practice because of the challenges of the COVID epidemic in addition to those of their typical practice environment [16].

Round the clock, 24-hour per day, shift-based work schedules necessitate that some healthcare personnel will work during individual circadian nadirs overnight and provoke fatigue [17]. Prior research indicates weariness and torpor most frequently and prominently manifest at 4 AM for shift workers, consistent with the notion that circadian rhythms of nocturnal workers impact fatigue along with shift duration [18]. Sleep deprivation hampers motor coordination, emotional IQ, and most importantly, reasoning cognition which combined result in inferior clinical performance [19, 20]. Exhaustion impairs reasoning comparable to alcohol intoxication; specifically, research has demonstrated that mental capacity deteriorates following 17-hours of intense cognition and wakefulness mimicking the impact

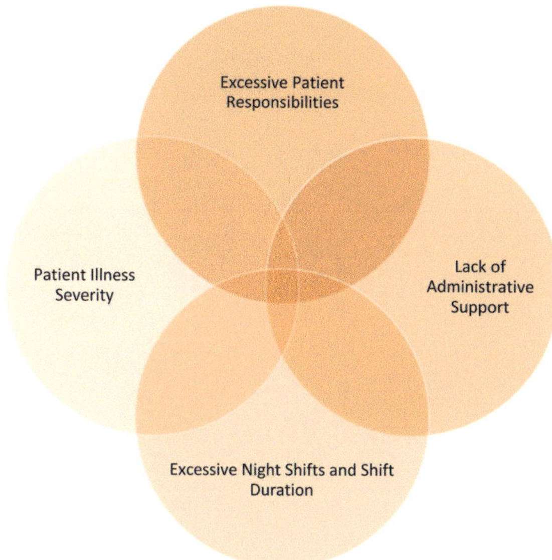

Figure 1.
Factors contributing to physician burnout.

of blood alcohol concentrations of 50 mg/dL [21]. The odds of reporting at least one fatigue related clinically significant medical miscue impacting patient safety and outcomes accrues by a factor of eight during months in which residents work five or more overnight shifts, in comparison to months in which they do not work overnight [22]. The relationship between onerous working hours, especially hours worked overnight, resulting in mental and physical exhaustion have disproportionately impacted physicians in training since the development of the residency training system decades ago [23]. In addition to impairing job performance and productivity, exhaustion escalates the risk of personal accidents and injuries of clinicians outside the hospital [23, 24]. Burnout is further exacerbated by the acuity and intensity of the clinical environment most notably emergency departments and critical care units during overnight shifts [25]. Job related burnout places the clinicians themselves at risk psychological, personal, and physical impairment (See **Figure 2**) [24]. Mental and physical fatigue increases the likelihood of occupational injuries in the work place such as body fluid exposures and motor vehicle accidents during transit home after long and/or overnight shifts [17].

In addition to the challenges of providing their patients with quality medical care through continuously enhancing their scientific knowledge and compassion, clinicians' ever expanding workplace responsibilities include but are not limited to maintenance of numerous certifications related to their specialties, incorporation of the complexities of new electronic health records, adhering increasingly stringent and complex regulatory guidelines, medical cost analysis, patient perceptions of satisfaction of medical care provided (Press Ganey scores), and undergoing progressively more stringent degrees of scrutiny related to adherence to quality of care metrics [4]. These factors individually and in combination impact the quality of patient care, physician productivity, physician retention within healthcare networks, income, mental duress, and contribute to burnout [8, 21]. Organizational challenges such as self-aggrandizing leadership conduct, unrealistic work load demands, inadequate allocation of resources in the clinical

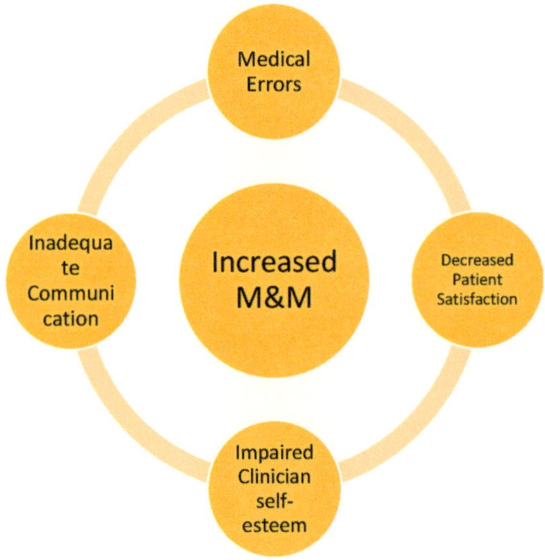

Figure 2.
Impact of physician burnout.

arena, substandard rewards, antagonistic interpersonal interactions, and insufficient opportunities for career advancement contribute to clinician dissatisfaction and erodes clinician morale [5]. Workplace and leadership inadequacy resulting in an inability to provide adequate, safe standards of care can be profoundly discouraging to physicians struggling to provide high quality, safe healthcare [12].

Recognizing the relationship between physician wellness and the safe, efficient functioning of healthcare organizations represents a crucial first step in confronting static health care workplace customs and culture that has heretofore been too reliant on physical stamina of the clinical workforce [16]. Medical staff including physicians must be part of a screening process for detection of burnout. A component of building a multimodal culture of wellness and healing to allay the development of burnout involves creating a culture in which healthcare providers can safely report mental anguish including feelings of burnout and have adequate access mental health care [6, 16]. Promoting physicians self-care can incorporate management of stress via mindfulness, talk therapy, physical activity, and meditation [8, 16, 22]. The Maslach Burnout Inventory (MBI), a self-reporting questionnaire for burnout screens three domains: emotional exhaustion, depersonalization, and depressed self-esteem [8]. Alternatively, the American Medical Association endorses the 10-item Zero Burnout Program for screening for emotional exhaustion [22], and has advocated for its five step process (research, measure, act, recognize, convene) to help guide physicians, care teams, and health system leaders on putting tactics and strategies to enhance practice productiveness, promote professional well-being, and move beyond burnout [8]. US governmental agencies including the US Surgeon General, the Centers for Disease Control and Prevention, the National Institute for Occupational Safety and Health have promoted efforts to support healthcare worker cognitive health and wellness [16].

Once burnout has been identified, expert opinion has advocated for a multifaceted strategy for treatment and deterrence utilizing individual and administrative tactics and strategies [8]. Documented correlations between burnout, exhaustion, and patient safety prompted the Institute of Medicine to recommend modifying physician trainee work hours to enhance wellness by decreasing shift duration, limiting incidence of overnight shifts, and safeguarding time off duty [11]. Brief naps during overnight shifts have correlated with enhanced wakefulness, comprehension, and recollection during overnight shifts especially in patient intense environments such as the intensive care unit and the emergency department [18]. Brief periods of exercise during shiftwork, especially overnight shifts, has correlated with improvement clinicians' mood and cognitive functioning [26]. Sage clinical leadership will incorporate medical staff's recommendations regarding reasonable workloads and in departmental functioning to enhance the clinicians' sense of support and team building thereby combating medical errors and improving clinical performance [14]. Encouraging mindfulness and team building, such as the patient-centered medical home provide physicians with emotional support and mentoring [22]. The medical home is a team focused healthcare administrative paradigm to provide comprehensive patient care through enhancing collaborative efforts. Colleagues, peers, and mentors provide role models and leadership to colleagues on how to prevent burnout and provide emotional support in the workplace to overcome work induced anxieties and depression [8].

3. Future directions

One of the challenges in assessing the impact of clinician burnout on patient safety is that much of the current research consists of subjective observational data and self-reported safety outcomes. Future investigations must focus on accounting for discrepancies between clinicians' perceptions of practice safety and quality in contrast to genuine objective assessment. Furthermore, scientific evaluation must examine the complex connections between clinicians and their working environments to further assess the relationship between burnout and patient safety [12]. Health worker burnout is not limited to individual physicians but also affects nurses, pharmacists, and other health professionals; because of its impact on health workers, it has the potential to impact the nation's health and economic security [6].

4. Conclusions

To address the growing recognition that physician welfare is an essential element of high-quality healthcare, methods and research must address physician and system level identification of, prevention of, and treatment of burnout [11]. Part of physician training and maintenance of certification must incorporate education about preventative techniques against emotional and physical exhaustion for individual physicians. On network and system levels, administrative and leadership management must strive to balance the needs of patients and physicians ensuring that clinicians are not overburdened in providing their best care, providing proper work and emotional support, ensuring quality interactions between providers, and support for providers in distress. Governmental and regulatory agencies can contribute meaningfully by providing regulations and standards to ensure both patient safety and prevention of excessive clinician responsibilities resulting in burnout.

Author details

Philip N. Salen[1*] and Stanislaw P. Stawicki[2]

1 Department of Emergency Medicine, St. Luke's University Health Network, Bethlehem, Pennsylvania, USA

2 Department of Research and Innovation, St. Luke's University Health Network, Bethlehem, Pennsylvania, USA

*Address all correspondence to: philipsalen@gmail.com

IntechOpen

© 2024 The Author(s). Licensee IntechOpen. This chapter is distributed under the terms of the Creative Commons Attribution License (http://creativecommons.org/licenses/by/3.0), which permits unrestricted use, distribution, and reproduction in any medium, provided the original work is properly cited.

References

[1] Slawomirski L, Auraaen A, Klazinga NS. The Economics of Patient Safety [Internet]. Organisation for Economic Co-Operation and Development (OECD) (OECD Health Working Papers). 2017. Available from: https://www.oecd-ilibrary.org/social-issues-migration-health/the-economics-of-patient-safety_5a9858cd-en

[2] Harris E, New CDC. Campaign targets health care worker burnout. JAMA. 2023;**330**(21):2044

[3] Busireddy KR, Miller JA, Ellison K, Ren V, Qayyum R, Panda M. Efficacy of interventions to reduce resident physician burnout: A systematic review. Journal of Graduate Medical Education. 2017;**9**(3):294-301

[4] Shanafelt TD, Dyrbye LN, West CP. Addressing physician burnout: The way forward. Journal of the American Medical Association. 2017;**317**(9):901-902

[5] Patel RS, Bachu R, Adikey A, Malik M, Shah M. Factors related to physician burnout and its consequences: A review. Behavioral Science. 2018;**8**(11). DOI: 10.3390/bs8110098

[6] Murthy VH. Confronting health worker burnout and well-being. The New England Journal of Medicine. 2022;**387**(7):577-579

[7] Dyrbye LN, Burke SE, Hardeman RR, Herrin J, Wittlin NM, Yeazel M, et al. Association of clinical specialty with symptoms of burnout and career choice regret among US resident physicians. Journal of the American Medical Association. 2018;**320**(11):1114-1130

[8] Mohanty D, Prabhu A, Lippmann S. Physician burnout: Signs and solutions. The Journal of Family Practice. 2019;**68**(8):442-446

[9] Tolentino JC, Guo WA, Ricca RL Jr, Vazquez D, Martins N, Sweeney J, et al. What's new in academic medicine: Can we effectively address the burnout epidemic in healthcare? International Journal of Academic Medicine. 2017;**3**(Suppl. 1):S1

[10] DeCaporale-Ryan L, Sakran JV, Grant SB, Alseidi A, Rosenberg T, Goldberg RF, et al. The undiagnosed pandemic: Burnout and depression within the surgical community. Current Problems in Surgery. 2017;**54**(9):453-502

[11] West CP, Dyrbye LN, Erwin PJ, Shanafelt TD. Interventions to prevent and reduce physician burnout: A systematic review and meta-analysis. Lancet. 2016;**388**(10057):2272-2281

[12] Weigl M. Physician burnout undermines safe healthcare. BMJ. 2022;**378**:o2157

[13] Dyrbye L, Shanafelt T. A narrative review on burnout experienced by medical students and residents. Medical Education. 2016;**50**(1):132-149

[14] Jarrar M, Al-Bsheish M, Albaker W, Alsaad I, Alkhalifa E, Alnufaili S, et al. Hospital work conditions and the mediation role of burnout: Residents and practicing physicians reporting adverse events. Risk Management Healthcare Policy. 2023;**16**:1-13

[15] West CP, Tan AD, Habermann TM, Sloan JA, Shanafelt TD. Association of resident fatigue and distress with perceived medical errors. Journal of the American Medical Association. 2009;**302**(12):1294-1300

[16] Kuehn BM. Physicians are more burned out than ever-here's what can be done about it. Journal of the American Medical Association. 2023;**329**(10):785-787

[17] Philibert I, Nasca T, Brigham T, Shapiro J. Duty-hour limits and patient care and resident outcomes: Can high-quality studies offer insight into complex relationships? Annual Review of Medicine. 2013;**64**:467-483

[18] McDonald J, Potyk D, Fischer D, Parmenter B, Lillis T, Tompkins L, et al. Napping on the night shift: A study of sleep, performance, and learning in physicians-in-training. Journal of Graduate Medical Education. 2013;**5**(4):634-638

[19] Osborne R, Parshuram CS. Delinking resident duty hours from patient safety. BMC Medical Education. 2014;**14**(Suppl. 1):S2

[20] Ntracha A, Iakovakis D, Hadjidimitriou S, Charisis VS, Tsolaki M, Hadjileontiadis LJ. Detection of mild cognitive impairment through natural language and touchscreen typing processing. Frontiers in Digital Health. 2020;**2**:567158

[21] Tait DR, Hatherill M, Van Der Meeren O, Ginsberg AM, Van Brakel E, Salaun B, et al. Final analysis of a trial of M72/AS01E vaccine to prevent tuberculosis. The New England Journal of Medicine. 2019. DOI: 10.1056/NEJMoa1909953

[22] Linzer M, Levine R, Meltzer D, Poplau S, Warde C, West CP. 10 bold steps to prevent burnout in general internal medicine. Journal of General Internal Medicine. 2014;**29**(1):18-20

[23] Blum AB, Shea S, Czeisler CA, Landrigan CP, Leape L. Implementing the 2009 Institute of Medicine recommendations on resident physician work hours, supervision, and safety. Nature and Science of Sleep. 2011;**3**:47-85

[24] West CP, Huschka MM, Novotny PJ, Sloan JA, Kolars JC, Habermann TM, et al. Association of perceived medical errors with resident distress and empathy: A prospective longitudinal study. Journal of the American Medical Association. 2006;**296**(9):1071-1078

[25] Hodkinson A, Zhou A, Johnson J, Geraghty K, Riley R, Zhou A, et al. Associations of physician burnout with career engagement and quality of patient care: Systematic review and meta-analysis. BMJ. 2022;**14**(378):e070442

[26] Philibert I. What is known: Examining the empirical literature in resident work hours using 30 influential articles. Journal of Graduate Medical Education. 2016;**8**(5):795-805

Chapter 2

Building a Safety-Centric Culture That Fosters Psychological Safety from Onboarding Onwards

Pablo Moreno Franco, LaRissa Adams, Sandy C. Booth and Grace M. Arteaga

Abstract

The healthcare system's evolution mirrors the Industrial Revolution, advancing from Healthcare 1.0's new economics and epidemics to Healthcare 2.0's mass production. With Healthcare 3.0, micro-controllers and computers revolutionized diagnostics and education, ushering in evidence-based medicine. Now, the healthcare sector is preparing to embrace Health 4.0, integrating digital technology, cyber-physical systems, and Artificial Intelligence (AI) for personalized, proactive care, marking a shift toward a more unified, efficient, patient-centric model. Yet, Health 4.0 introduces risks like cybersecurity and ethical dilemmas, necessitating a culture of safety and human connection as a cornerstone within healthcare organizations. This chapter outlines how healthcare entities can become high-reliability organizations (HROs) and adept at navigating complex, risky environments to maintain high safety and performance standards by preempting threats. It delves into Safety 2.0, which focuses on learning from successes to enhance HRO practices. Emphasizing humble leadership and trust, the chapter highlights psychological safety's role in fostering open communication, teamwork, and innovation. It offers guidance for integrating new staff and establishing safety norms in Health 4.0. Aimed at healthcare leaders, managers, and staff, this chapter provides insights into improving service safety, quality, and mental well-being in the sector.

Keywords: healthcare, safety, leadership, psychological safety, high-reliability organizations, communication, trust, artificial intelligence, patient experience, virtual work

1. Introduction

Healthcare has undergone significant changes in recent years, particularly after the changes created during the SARS-CoV-2 pandemic, which have sped up the digital transformation of the industry with the emergence of Health 4.0 and the use of artificial intelligence (AI) in patient care [1, 2]. Creating a culture that supports open communication, psychological safety, and continuous learning is vital for organizations to prioritize the safety and well-being of their employees in this context. In this chapter, we will explore the critical components of a culture focused on safety and provide helpful advice for building and maintaining such a culture in the workplace.

2. Method

This chapter is based on a literature review of the current trends and challenges in healthcare safety, focusing on high reliability, adapting to new technology, and continuing learning. We followed a systematic search strategy to identify relevant sources from academic databases, government publications, and industry-related websites. The search terms included single and paired combinations of the following keywords: Healthcare, Safety, Leadership, Psychological Safety, High-Reliability Organizations, Safety huddles, Communication, Trust, Technology, AI, Quality, Patient Experience, and Virtual Work. We used PubMed, MEDLINE, and Google™ Scholar as the main search engines. We applied filters for language (English), publication date (2010–2024), and document type (peer-reviewed articles, reports, guidelines, white papers, and books). We also scanned the reference lists of the selected sources to find additional relevant literature. We excluded articles that were not relevant to healthcare and were not in English. The themes extracted from the literature review were discussed among the authors and with professional colleagues with leadership and patient safety expertise. They served as the foundation for the main topics covered in this chapter.

2.1 The new normal in healthcare: the 'patient's perspective

2.1.1 Family involvement in patient care

Families face extreme uncertainty when their loved ones are admitted to the hospital, particularly to an Intensive Care Unit (ICU) setting [3]. There is a sense of loss of control, which is enhanced by physical transformation noted in their family members, and it is particularly stressful when there are complications and extended stays [4]. The angst the families encounter is heightened when infection control measures are required to protect family and health staff members [5].

Involving family members in health care relies on active participation in the care and decision-making process and support of the patient's family. In healthcare settings, involving family members can significantly benefit the patient and the healthcare team [6, 7]. Family members can provide emotional support to the patient, improving their overall well-being and aiding their recovery. Additionally, family members often play a crucial role in advocating for the patient's needs and preferences. They also serve as a bridge between the patient and the healthcare team, helping to ensure that essential and valuable information is effectively communicated and understood by the healthcare providers. They can also help clarify medical information and provide context about the patient's health history. In outpatient settings, family members can aid in coordinating care, ensure that the patient receives necessary medications, has adequate appointments, and understands treatment plans. When the patient is unable to make their own medical decision, family members can serve as surrogate decision-makers, advocating for the patient's best interest and ensuring that their wishes are respected [8].

Healthcare providers must recognize and respect the valuable emotional support that family members can provide in caring for their loved ones and actively involve them in the appropriate processes. Effective communication, collaboration, and partnership between healthcare professionals and family members can contribute to better outcomes and overall satisfaction with the care received [9].

2.1.2 Visitation limitations

Patient Experience: Patient visitation from family in the healthcare setting refers to the practice of allowing family members or loved ones to visit and spend time with the patient who is receiving medical care in a hospital or healthcare facility where visitation policies can vary depending on the specific healthcare institution, the patient's condition, and any infection control measures that may be in place [10].

There are several vital purposes to allow for visitation: family members provide emotional comfort and support to the patient, which can positively impact their well-being and recovery. They also advocate for the patient, sharing that their needs and concerns are addressed and communicating their preferences to the healthcare team. They also can serve as facilitators between the patient and the healthcare team, providing valuable information on medical history, needs, and patient preferences.

Visitation policies may have specific guidelines regarding the number of visitors allowed, visiting hours, and any restrictions based on the patient's condition or the particular unit within the healthcare facility. In some cases, such as during a pandemic, visitation policies may be more restrictive to ensure the safety of the patient, staff, and visitors [11].

Overall, patient visitation from family members is recognized as an essential aspect of patient-centered care, and healthcare institutions strive to balance the benefits of visitation with the need to maintain a safe and healing environment. It is vital for healthcare providers to communicate visitation policies clearly to patients and their families and to accommodate visitation whenever possible to support the patient's well-being [12].

2.1.3 Patient experience

Patient experience refers to all patient exchanges with the healthcare system, including their perceptions, interactions, and overall satisfaction with the care they receive. It encompasses every aspect of the patient's journey, from scheduling appointments and registration to delivering care, discharge process, and follow-up care [13, 14].

Essential aspects of patient experience include the effectiveness of communication between healthcare providers, staff, and patients, including the clarity of information provided, active listening, and respectful dialog. It is also influenced by the ease of scheduling appointments, waiting times, access to different specialists, and the availability of resources and services. The quality of care provided for the patient includes the technical quality of the medical treatment, the success of interventions, the attention to safety and infection control, and the overall care outcome. The physical environment also plays a significant role in significantly impacting the 'patient's experience, including cleanliness, comfort, privacy, and amenities [15]. A crucial factor related to the patient's experience is the ability of healthcare providers to demonstrate empathy, compassion, understanding, and emotional support for the patient's needs and concerns. The 'patient's perception of empathy and compassion in their medical care is the foundation of trust in the medical system. Creating trust allows patients to actively become involved in their care, including sharing- decision-making, involvement in care planning, and believing they receive accurate and educated information about their condition and treatment options [16, 17].

Healthcare systems prioritize patient experience because it has been shown to directly impact health outcomes, patient safety, and overall patient satisfaction. Patient experience is increasingly recognized as an essential component of high-quality care delivery, and it's often measured through patient satisfaction surveys, feedback mechanisms, and other tools to capture the patient's perspective [18]. Improving patient experience requires a focus on patient-centered care, active engagement, and continuous efforts to enhance the overall quality of care delivery. Extensive reviews of the literature have described interventions that improve the patient experience, including developing support groups including social workers, psychological professionals, and nursing groups, clinician training, journal writing by the families and patients, face-to-face meetings for medical updates, family participation during medical rounds, open visiting hours, information to families through nursing staff, pamphlets, use of technology (DVDs, phones, SMS (Short Message Service), developing family care plans, and improving the physical environment [6].

2.2 The new normal in healthcare: the healthcare 'provider's perspective

2.2.1 Staff shortages

During the COVID-19 pandemic and afterward, staff shortages have significantly impacted medical care [19]. The increased demand for healthcare services due to the pandemic exacerbated staffing issues and created additional challenges for the healthcare industry. Beyond the COVID-19 pandemic, the healthcare industry continues to be challenged, needing experienced healthcare providers. A decrease in the quality of care with staff shortages reduces the patient-healthcare provider interface and decreases time dedicated to each patient. During limited nurse staffing, there is an increased risk of adverse events, poor patient experience, and reduced treatment effectiveness [20]. Staff shortages can also affect the timing of test results and the procedures required, potentially delaying patient diagnosis and treatment and theoretically increasing patient safety events [21]. The effects of staff shortages continue as healthcare systems work to rebuild their workforce after the SARS-CoV-2 pandemic and address the long-term impacts on staff mental health and well-being. Solutions to address this issue have been documented since the pandemic's beginning, addressing mutual support and communication [22].

2.2.2 Workforce demoralization

The shortage of medical staff results in healthcare workers being overworked and experiencing burnout, negatively impacting patient care [23]. Aiken et al. found a strong association between high patient-to-nurse ratios, higher emotional exhaustion, and greater job dissatisfaction. There was also a significant impact on morbidity and mortality among the surgical patients included in the study. Further investigations have associated the shortage of nursing staff with a negative effect on patient safety [24]. Several investigators have noted a correlation between perceived medical errors and burnout [25, 26]. There can be an increased perception of medical errors since the providers cannot deliver the care required under normal circumstances [27]. Tawfik et al. described in a cross-sectional study how burnout, well-being, and work unit safety were strongly and independently associated with perceived medical errors [28]. Further, in a prospective study of self-perceived medical errors among internal medicine residents, burnout predicted subsequent perceived medical errors and could be related in a reciprocal cycle [29].

Job experience – An essential outcome of COVID-19 was the revelation of healthcare systems working under already stressed systems, which led to a job-related crisis. System stresses, overwork, and poor working conditions further exacerbated workforce strain, under-staffing, and high job turnover rates [30]. Burnout is an occupational phenomenon characterized by 1) fatigue or exhaustion, 2) negative feelings towards 'one's job, and 3) reduced professional efficacy [31].

Mental and emotional Health - During and in the post-pandemic period, mental well-being became and continues to be a significant priority. It became clear that not addressing mental and emotional health creates a significant societal financial burden with a notable impact on the healthcare community and causes higher rates of mental disorders and psychological distress [32]. In 2019, a consensus from the National Academies of Sciences, Engineering, and Medicine proposed a systems model of clinician burnout that emphasizes not only targeting downstream interventions (meditation as an example) but emphasizing the importance of systematic solutions considered upstream interventions (improving the product of the work environment) [31]. In this report, the authors call for increased investment in research and policy changes supporting novel solutions, emphasizing upstream solutions, including changes in government and insurance policies, EMR redesign, and training professionals in norms and expectations.

High-Performing Teams - Enhanced teamwork and teaming: At the highest peak of the pandemic, healthcare providers started to adapt to new challenges with increased collaboration: nurses and respiratory therapists integrated with laboratory services, and primary care physicians worked with intensivists. During this challenging time, the medical community embraced this challenge by supporting each other, learning to adapt during a medical crisis, breaking down hierarchy levels, and supporting each other [22, 33].

2.3 Creating a service excellence culture

2.3.1 Components of high-reliability organizations

High-reliability organizations (HROs) are identified as industries with a high risk of safety events and personal harm due to the catastrophic consequences that can occur when something goes wrong. HROs include the airline industry, nuclear power plants, and healthcare. These industries include extraordinarily complex processes with interdependent relationships that require strong teamwork. When a process fails, the results are commonly loss of life. Understanding the significance of the loss of life, these organizations must be highly reliable in everything related to safety. Therefore, HROs have become fixated on the risk of failure and how to prevent failure. Through investigations into significant accidents and events, organizations have learned there is always an element of awareness before the accident, so organizations are now focused on learning to identify these risks and then mitigating those risks to prevent the incident [34].

The Joint Commission identifies three pillars of high-reliability organizations as

i. Leadership committed to zero harm

ii. Safety Culture

iii. Robust Process Improvement® (RPI) [35].

HROs must begin with the first pillar of these three pillars, a leadership committed to zero harm. Leadership must be committed to zero harm and possess the characteristics required to build trust with the staff and throughout the organization. Building trust can be challenging and will take time. Trust is simply consistency over time. When staff consistently see leadership engaged, listening, and responding, they will begin to believe that leadership is committed to zero harm and supporting the staff.

One method to measure if staff trust leaders is through reporting. This component is part of the second pillar, a safety culture. All HROs must have a reporting system that allows staff to share events and, more importantly, report possible hazards or unsafe conditions. For an organization to become highly reliable, it must move from reactive to proactive. This approach can only be accomplished when leaders listen to the frontline providers [36]. It also means including members who designed all processes and were aware of unsafe conditions and failures. Some refer to this situation as the 'black swans." This term denotes the black swans on the west coast of Australia that were unknown to the Europeans before they visited this location. While the Aboriginal people were always aware of the black swans, outsiders did not even know of their existence. This metaphor applies to an HRO; if leaders do not know risks exist, they are not listening to those who are aware of them. So, one could theorize that all events are preventable if leaders only talk to the right people [37].

This preamble leads to the third pillar of robust process improvement. Since the 'To Err is Human: Building a Safer Health 'System' publication in 1999, healthcare has embraced quality improvement methodologies. However, acknowledging the methodologies is not enough. The organization must implement the known best practices of change management, lean methodology, and six sigma. Robust Process Improvement (RPI®) is a blended set of strategies, tools, methods, and training programs incorporating all three best-known practices to improve clinical outcomes and business processes. Of these three, "change management" is defined as a systematic way to implement and sustain good solutions, and it is the one component that can prevent the sustainment of any improvement, particularly if people do not easily accept, or even resist, good solutions regardless of their intentions. Dr. Chassin, President of the Joint Commission, stated, "Process improvement in healthcare 'isn't rocket science. It's much more difficult than that because rocket science involves getting machines to behave as you want them to. With process improvement, you have to change the behavior of people" [35].

Process improvement also includes an effective communication network to ensure sustainable control plans, close the communication loop to all stakeholders [38], and a repository of lessons learned to prevent repeat occurrences. This approach addresses complex problem-solving with a systematic, data-driven approach.

To become proactive, an organization needs leaders who can build trust with staff and encourage them to report all risks. However, the reports must be accompanied by feedback to the staff who reported them. This feedback and loop-closure is the only way to ensure the reporters witness improvement. The reporting system is the life cycle of an HRO: *trust, report, improve,* as demonstrated in **Figure 1** [39]. Without improvement and communication circled back to staff, each unanswered report will erode the trust that someone will respond. Over time, the lack of trust will erode the culture of the organization, and the element of high reliability will be lost.

The healthcare setting has become a complex environment where operations are high-risk and require highly effective solutions and high interdependence of various aspects of organizational performance to prevent failure. HROs are mindful organizations that place significant effort into developing a culture of constant awareness of the possibility of failure. This culture leads to "collective mindfulness," where all workers look for and report minor problems or unsafe conditions, preventing severe events [39]. Five basic principles characterizing an HRO can be divided into two groups: 1) anticipatory action and 2) containment. These two major groups have been described graphically in **Figure 2**. Both groups place patient safety as the framework with which to work. The anticipatory action includes a. preoccupation with failure consisting of driving a culture to zero harm and addressing minimal risks or events; b. reluctance to simplify by striving to understand all events and diving into the root causes to find solutions; c. sensitivity to operations by being conscious of strong correlations between people, processes, and systems impacting the outcome.

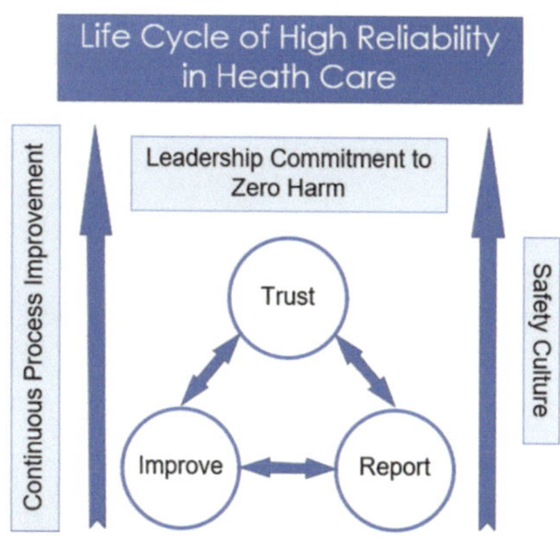

Figure 1.
The life cycle of high reliability begins with building trust that encourages reporting of events and unsafe conditions. That reporting leads to improvement, reinforcing trust. This life cycle supports the commitment to zero harm by having a safety culture and continuous process improvement.

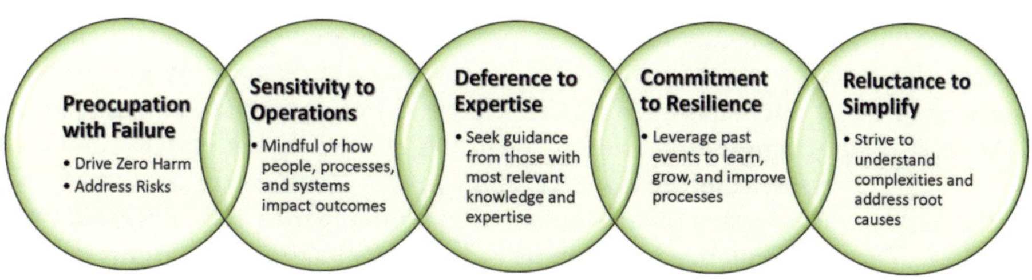

Figure 2.
High-reliability organization (HRO.) principles. The five principles of organizational mindfulness are the core of HROs. These fundamental principles include anticipation (preoccupation with failure, reluctance to simplify, sensitivity to operations) and containment (commitment to resilience and deference to expertise) [40].

The containment actions include a. commitment to resilience, where past events are used to learn, grow, and improve processes to improve the system; and b.deference to expertise, where insights from staff with pertinent safety knowledge are embraced.

2.3.2 Introducing human connection

Virtual health care requires effective and compassionate human connection for quality health care delivery [41]. Several research-based tips for enhancing human connection in the virtual healthcare setting have been described by Cooley et al. [42]. Some recommendations include A. Being present; demonstrating focus, interest, and curiosity; reducing distractions and interruptions during virtual interactions; B. Identifying needs; asking open-ended questions and finding preferences and expectations, goals, and priorities; C. Listening; attending to verbal and nonverbal signals, reflecting, recapping main points, and verifying understanding; D. Responding with empathy; recognizing and affirming emotions, expressing support and compassion, and giving hope and reassurance; E. Sharing information; providing clear, brief, and relevant information, using simple language and visual aids, and encouraging questions and feedback.

These tips can help improve the personal quality of virtual communication by video or phone and can be helpful for patients and colleagues. Furthermore, other sources recommend balancing digital innovation and human connection by incorporating personal interaction in health care, such as developing a human-centered culture that values and rewards personal connection and collaboration [43]. Using technology to enhance, not substitute, human abilities and relationships. Offering training and support for health care providers and patients to use virtual health technologies efficiently and comfortably [41].

2.3.3 From H.R.O. To culture of safety

a. Tangible to front healthcare staff

b. Resonance of practice on a day-to-day label

c. Technology in the new workforce

d. Difference in mindset and understanding in communication in the new generations

e. Tread of technology

Understanding how technology has helped and hindered current healthcare practices is critical for healthcare leaders [44]. With the current workforce growing up with technology, there has been a disruption in the expression of empathy and an alteration in society's communication patterns [45]. Given that effective, emotionally intelligent conversations are not natural for people, training for the workforce with the behaviors necessary to develop emotional intelligence and digital empathy [46]. The leaders are challenged to support safety while balancing accountability through a fair and just culture. This gap in quality is countered by the emergence of AI to aid in the level of excellence while fostering more effective and efficient delivery of patient care. Conversely, the older, more experienced staff are comfortable with the soft skills of personal interactions and feedback. This leaves leadership with the blend of the younger workforce with the technical skills to support the emergence of AI technology and the older workforce with the soft skills of human interactions to support teamwork.

The other factor of technology now included in healthcare is the ever-growing population of virtual staff [47]. Team building activities with virtual staff are a requirement to ensure safety and job satisfaction [48].

2.3.4 Humanizing back-2-basics: reverting to foundational best practices. Machines do not care. People care

a. Onboarding Process and Expectations

The SARS-CoV-2 pandemic forced organizations to convert to a virtual onboarding process to quickly get staff to a productive status [49]. While this provided timing flexibility and increased efficiency, it also reduced the efficacy of onboarding for a safety culture. In health care, the primary factor is human interaction. In an organization based on human interaction, removing that interaction prevents the organization from setting proper expectations for its safety culture.

From the first day of employment, the organization is responsible for providing professional behavior expectations, compliance with policies, and establishing a fair and just culture. It is not easy to convey the significance of these expectations without solid communication [36]. These expectations were established as best practices years before the availability of virtual options [47]. Organizations must return to at least some portion of onboarding occurring in a face-to-face setting if leadership desires the ingrained safety culture necessary to prevent harm [50].

b. Safety behaviors

Safety is the cornerstone of healthcare facilities. A safe environment requires identifying behaviors demonstrating professional ethics and the organization's culture and environment [36]. These behaviors should be established at each organization according to the mission and values of the organization. Additionally, the behaviors should be universal to clinical and non-clinical staff. Some examples of safe behaviors include paying attention to detail, speaking up, being respectful, and supporting each other. Each of these behaviors applies to all roles within the organization and contributes to preventing safety errors. The 'leadership's behavior directly indicates the organization's safety culture. If the 'leader's attitude includes blaming or excessive questioning, the safety culture will diminish, and an environment of fear will grow [36].

Thus, it is essential to adopt safety behaviors that will be timeless. Staff are most successful when the expectations are set and do not frequently change. This approach applies to behaviors in the work environment. When professionalism is established during the onboarding process, it is easy to sustain that level. It becomes much more challenging to correct unwanted behaviors that have been allowed.

As discussed later in the chapter, leadership must balance safety with accountability. Senior staff members should clearly show expectations of behavior and accountability to new members starting the first day of employment. It is critical to identify the appropriate response when expectations are not met. This approach is considered accountability, not punishment. Having a candid conversation and providing feedback is more valuable and productive than lighthearted comments [51]. However, if staff are not aware of expectations or the response plan when these expectations are not met, accountability can feel punitive. High levels of psychological safety, as evidenced by transparent conversations, increased safety reporting, and surveys, resulting in a safety culture, will prevent this feeling for staff.

c. Communication

When discussing communication as a best practice, we must identify the essential components of communication. Those include speaking and listening. Inherently, people will communicate with confidence on topics of familiarity. Some speak well in individual conversations, while others are confident in a group. In either case, it is the responsibility of the speaker and listener to share information. Speakers need to use clear and concise language. Listeners need to have the psychological safety to speak up.

Challenges for speakers and listeners can range from terminology to culture to learned behaviors. Communication skills can be improved with the appropriate level of emotional intelligence. When a speaker can recognize the listener's facial expressions and body language, they can adjust the conversation to ensure comprehension. This communication can be accomplished through sincere questions or pausing to allow the listener to speak up. At this moment, the responsibility shifts to the listener to identify whether the information is incomplete or lacks understanding. Active listening is a familiar concept. However, active listening is not sufficient to foster effective communication. The listener needs to go beyond and listen to understand. When all the people in a conversation are listening to understand instead of just absorbing the content, there is an increase in the efficacy of the conversation [51].

One might think that all organizations are proficient in communication since it is a fundamental skill. Often, safety incidents are caused by communication problems. Improving communication can significantly reduce incidents and enhance safety [52].

d. Handoff

To achieve HRO status, complex organizations need effective collaboration among their teams. When considering handoffs in that context, a strong team's primary function is to provide effective handoffs to maintain a level of excellence and continuity [53]. Many of the HROs provide services that operate all day hours, requiring the team to transition from one shift to another consistently. Additionally, complex work requires handoffs between stakeholders for diverse types of work, including projects, proposals, improvements, etc. This essential component of work should not be assumed or overlooked. To have an effective handoff, the teammates must be intentional and mindful and operate with a level of standardization that will provide a firm foundation of operations.

When handoffs are incomplete or poorly facilitated, the consequences can be catastrophic. Imagine the medication being delivered incorrectly, the inclement weather notice affecting the flight patterns not being shared, or the equipment malfunction that changed the nuclear power level but was not communicated. Any of these events could have been prevented with an effective handoff. Remember that an effective handoff requires articulate communication and techniques to ensure a good handoff. These techniques include the teach-back method, following up with a written form to verbal communication, or utilizing checklists during the handoff. Implementing a standardized method of the handoff process reduces the risk of error [53].

e. Mutual Support

Mutual support may be considered one of the safe behaviors an organization would like to identify as an expectation. While support may seem obvious, this type of support is not simply being kind to your colleagues but developing a spirit of teamwork that transcends getting the job done. As technology continues to emerge, we know the human component of most organizations will continue to be the greatest resource. As such, humans instinctively need to belong and feel valued by their organizations and teams.

It is essential to recognize that a component of psychological safety is learning to be vulnerable and take interpersonal risks to speak up. Mutual support is what allows someone to take that risk. Colleagues must feel heard and understood about the topic and their feelings [51]. When someone feels supported, they can learn, test possibilities, and grow in their work environment, leading to job satisfaction and longevity within the organization.

Figure 3 summarizes the fundamental best practices described, which detail the onboarding, clearly identified expected behaviors and establishment of a fair and just culture aiming for effective teamwork.

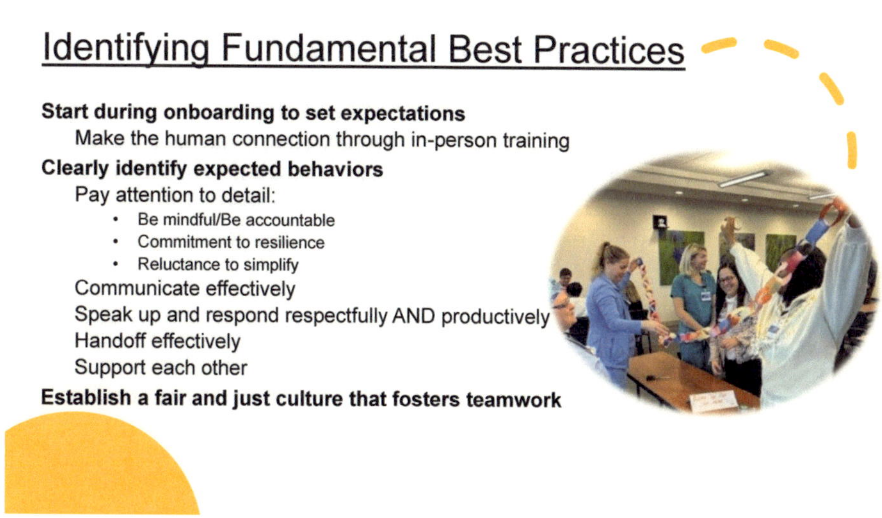

Figure 3.
In-person training creates a human connection among teams and the organization. Setting expectations and articulating the components of the professional environment supports new staff. Establishing a fair and just culture will encourage and promote a teaming environment.

2.3.5 From the beginning: safety huddles

How safety huddles started in healthcare

Safety huddles are short, daily gatherings where frontline staff and leaders talk about safety concerns and exchange information. They improve communication, collaboration, and problem-solving across units and departments and foster a safe culture and continuous learning [54, 55].

The origin of safety huddles can be traced back to the aviation industry, where crew members gather before each flight to review the flight plan, weather conditions, potential risks, and contingency plans [56–58]. This practice was adopted by other high-risk industries, such as nuclear power, military, and firefighting, to enhance situational awareness and prevent errors.

Safety huddles in healthcare originated in the intensive care unit (ICU) setting, where they helped to manage care transfers, track patient conditions, and detect safety risks [59]. The advantages of safety huddles include improved teamwork, reduced length of stay, lower mortality rates, and fewer adverse events [60].

Safety huddles gradually expanded to other clinical settings and layers of the organization, from hospital units and offices to health centers and health systems [59]. Safety huddles became essential to patient safety programs and quality improvement efforts, such as the Institute for Healthcare Improvement's 100,000 Lives Campaign and the World Health Organization's Surgical Safety Checklist [61].

Safety huddles have become a familiar and effective way to improve patient safety and quality of care in healthcare settings. They allow staff to exchange information, voice issues, learn from mistakes, and acknowledge achievements. They also let leaders hear from frontline workers, give feedback, and distribute resources. Safety huddles can help build a positive and supportive work environment where staff feel appreciated, respected, and enabled [59, 62, 63].

a. The use of scripts

Scripts are helpful for safety huddles, as they help maintain consistency and efficiency in meetings. Scripts offer a structured huddle format, which can help participants remain focused and on track [64]. They also help ensure that all critical topics get discussed and everyone has a chance to participate. Scripts can be created locally and adapted to the organization's specific needs [65]. They usually include a concise introduction, a review of safety concerns, a discussion of any recent incidents or near-misses, and any action items from previous huddles [66]. With the use of scripts, safety huddles can be more successful in finding and resolving safety issues, enhancing teamwork, and fostering a culture of safety.

b. Efficiency and effectiveness

Safety huddles can improve the efficiency and effectiveness of communication, collaboration, and problem-solving among healthcare teams. A recent article states that safety huddles are an effective way for healthcare teams to communicate, evaluate their performance, prevent safety issues before they happen, hold each other accountable, and ensure that safety measures are embedded in the system [59]. Huddles involve and motivate frontline staff in finding problems and create a culture of teamwork and quality, which helps to provide safer care [67]. Huddles have improved patient safety in various areas such as wrong-site surgery, medication errors, poor hand hygiene, unrecognized clinical deterioration, serious safety events, and near misses [66]. Huddles enhance individual and collective responsibility for patient safety, set a regular time during the workday or shift to focus on care coordination, enable quick and direct clarification of issues, reduce distractions during the rest of the workday, and support a culture of empowerment and collaboration in healthcare teams [55].

Data sharing

Data sharing is a crucial part of safety huddles in healthcare. Lamming, Montague, Crosswaite et al. describe how safety huddles can help prevent and resolve safety issues related to electronic health records [68]. The authors describe how safety huddles can be a valuable strategy to identify and mitigate safety concerns and improve teamwork. By sharing data during safety huddles, healthcare teams can identify potential safety hazards, track progress, and develop targeted interventions to improve patient safety and quality of care. This group recommends adjusting safety huddle fidelity criteria to include factors most valuable by frontline staff. describes the main content discussed during safety huddles.

c. Ownership, accountability, and leadership

Safety huddles in healthcare require ownership, accountability, and leadership presence. The Washington State Hospital Association suggests that leaders from different hospital or health system departments gather daily to share what happened in the last 24 hours and decide what actions are needed to address critical safety issues [55]. Safety huddles help ensure leaders are aware of safety concerns and accountable for addressing them (**Table 1**). Ownership of safety huddles can be shared among frontline staff and leaders, with each member taking responsibility for identifying and addressing safety concerns. One of the key factors that can enhance the effectiveness of safety huddles is leadership presence. However, leadership presence does not mean leaders should dominate or direct the safety huddle. Instead, leaders should act as facilitators, supporters, and role models for staff, encouraging open and honest communication, feedback, and problem-solving.

Data Type	Description
Patient safety incidents	Discuss any patient safety incidents since the last huddle, including near-misses, falls, medication errors, and other adverse events.
Staffing levels	Reviewing staffing levels and identifying potential staffing issues that could impact patient safety.
Equipment and supplies	Discuss equipment or supply issues impacting patient care, such as malfunctioning equipment or low inventory levels.
Infection control	Reviewing infection control practices and identifying any potential issues or concerns.
Patient flow	Discuss patient flow and identify any bottlenecks or delays that could impact patient safety or quality of care.
Quality metrics	Review quality metrics, such as readmission rates, patient satisfaction scores, and compliance with clinical guidelines.
Staff training	Discuss staff training needs and identify gaps in knowledge or skills that could impact patient safety.

Table 1.
Safety huddles in healthcare.

d. Closing the loop

Creating systems to close the loop and communicate with staff about how the issues discussed are addressed is paramount [55]. It is recommended that healthcare organizations use multiple Excellence Canada, it is recommended that healthcare organizations use multiple mechanisms to transfer learning from the analysis between care units through memos, storytelling, huddles, team-based peer review rounds, journal clubs, patient safety workshops using case-based learning methods, and newsletters (**Table 2**).

Leaders should also demonstrate their commitment to patient safety by following up on action items, providing resources and support, and recognizing and rewarding good practices. By having leadership presence in safety huddles, healthcare teams can ensure that safety concerns are addressed promptly and effectively and that everyone is accountable for patient safety (**Table 3**).

Share what was learned internally	
Share what was learned from the analysis with internal stakeholders	• Identify the key stakeholders who need to be informed of the outcomes, such as patients, families, staff, managers, and external agencies.
	• Determine the best mode and timing of communication, such as face-to-face, phone, email, or written reports, and consider the urgency, sensitivity, and confidentiality of the information
	• Communicate the analysis findings to internal stakeholders to ensure they are aware and can share their input.
Interface recommended actions	• Provide clear and accurate information about what happened, why it happened, what actions were taken, and what changes were implemented or planned to prevent recurrence.
	• Communicate recommended actions to all stakeholders,
	• Invite questions and feedback from the stakeholders, and listen empathically to their concerns, emotions, and suggestions
Communicate results of recommended actions	• Document the communication process and outcomes and report any unresolved issues or new learning to the appropriate authority or committee.
Engage with the patient/family in this process	Sharing stories can foster trust, learning, and change among staff and leaders, and promote a culture of safety and transparency.
	• Respect the patient/family's wishes and preferences about sharing personal or confidential information and get their permission and consent first.
	• Discuss the pros and cons of sharing experiences, such as enhancing learning, influencing policy, providing feedback, increasing empathy, or triggering emotions.
	• Support and resource the patient/family to share their experiences in several ways, such as storytelling, surveys, interviews, focus groups, committees, or events.
	• Thank and appreciate the patient/family for their courage and contribution in sharing their experiences and update them on the outcomes and impacts of their sharing.

Share what was learned internally	
Communicate what has been implemented and the results	• Review the recommended actions, their status, and their impact. Maintain transparency and trust by being honest if plans have changed and sharing why.
Use multiple mechanisms that transfer learning from the analysis between care units	• Follow the organizational policies: use various methods that share the learning from the analysis across care units such as memos, storytelling, huddles, team-based peer review rounds, journal clubs, patient safety workshops using case-based learning methods and newsletters.
Maintain a record of communication	• Keep track of communication to make sure all relevant stakeholders are informed.
Recognize that sharing is a dialog	• Acknowledge that sharing is a conversation (not a one-sided transfer of information) and is continuous (more than once). Promote respectful, transparent communication about the outcomes of the incident analysis at all levels of the organization.
Share what was learned externally	
Use alerts, advisories, and repositories	• Explain the situation, causes and reasons, steps followed, and outcomes.
Develop an external communication plan	• Communicating to the public the steps taken, their results, pertinent background, and context information, and respecting the patient/family's preferences for sharing or not sharing their viewpoint
Prepare staff and the patient/family	• Consult with the staff and the patient/family beforehand about what, when, and how information will be communicated.

Table 2.
Proposed closing-the-loop strategies.

Analyze multiple incidents to find out common system problems.
Check if the lessons learned can be transferred to other processes in the organization.
Report any significant risks and/or best practices to senior leadership or other relevant committees.
Integrate findings with those from other systems to help reveal themes/patterns and speed up learning.
Evaluate the incident management process to find out strengths and areas for improvement, considering the analysis time, the quality and efficiency of the suggested actions, organizational guidance and supporting structures, communication, and processes for spreading the learning, and the experience of those who participated in the incident and the analysis.
Supporting Research and Innovation. Encourage and facilitate research and innovation projects that aim to learn from incidents and improve patient safety.

Table 3.
Expanding the role of safety leaders' involvement in safety huddles.

2.4 Leadership and psychological safety

2.4.1 Leadership characteristics and humility

Leadership and psychological safety are critical components of a healthy and productive work environment. According to a Frontiers in Psychology article [69], unpretentious leadership can positively influence follower attitudes and behaviors, such as job satisfaction, psychological empowerment, and engagement. The study explores the relationship between unpretentious leadership and follower creativity. It describes that psychological safety is critical in linking unpretentious leadership and follower creativity. This finding is consistent with most of the previous work that shows the mediating influence of psychological safety on the relationship between leadership and psychological safety [70].

A study explores the relationship between baseline leader humility and team psychological safety by examining the roles of humility variability and attractor strength. The study found that consistency reinforces, while inconsistency weakens, the effect of leader-expressed humility on team psychological safety. The findings also reveal that self-other agreement relates to the consistency of leader-expressed humility, depending on the level at which the (dis)agreement occurs. The study indicates that the results of unpretentious leadership rely on the leader's level of humility, how stable his/her humility is, and how powerful the attractor is [71].

2.4.2 Behaviors associated with building trust

As previously stated, trust is a critical component of the life cycle of a high-reliability organization. That trust must start with the leaders and be built through the staff to maintain a safe culture. Leadership styles vary, and while variation can bring richness to the organization, certain behaviors must be embraced to elicit trust. Servant or ethical leadership are terms used to describe these behaviors. Operating with sincerity, integrity, and compassion are all servant and ethical leadership elements. While transformational leadership is visionary in moving the organization forward, elevating the needs of the staff above themselves is a key marker of a servant or ethical leader. Combined with balanced and fair decision-making, it will build trust within the organization. Staff must feel the leaders are concerned about their well-being and genuinely have good intentions to support them [72], and can be demonstrated through transparent communication, investment of resources to help the staff, or personally engaging with the staff without a predetermined agenda. Leadership must be visible and approachable. By feeling connected to leadership, staff are intrinsically motivated to perform and remain engaged.

2.4.3 Components of psychological safety

Psychological safety in the work environment is where all staff feel comfortable expressing themselves by sharing ideas, concerns, and mistakes. This feeling comes from having confidence they will not be humiliated, punished, or blamed when speaking up [73]. Psychological safety creates transparency in communication and operations, which is critical to a high-reliability organization (HRO). The healthcare industry is a prime example of an HRO. In healthcare, the staff must be able to speak up to prevent medical errors. Two major types of errors are errors of omission that occur as a result of actions not taken, and errors that occur because of the wrong action taken [74]. These two examples illustrate the necessity of having a safety culture that embodies psychological safety.

The challenge is in creating and sustaining a culture of safety. HRO senior leadership has long understood the importance of a safety culture and its impact on the work environment, patient outcomes, and quality of care. However, permeating that understanding throughout the 'organization's workforce is challenging. With the advancement of technology, our workforce has become more accustomed to electronic communication versus face-to-face interactions. While efficient, this type of communication erodes the humanity of relationships, investing in those relationships and maintaining a skillset to support psychological safety in professional relationships. Yet these components are precisely what is needed to have psychological safety. Conversations are the cornerstone of an organizational culture. One can ascertain the organization's psychological safety level by listening to conversations among colleagues. Because psychological safety is being able to speak candidly, leaders and staff must have more than just sharing information. Leaders must understand their staff members' emotions, values, and attitudes that pertain to daily work and respond accordingly [51]. Active listening is no longer adequate for creating psychological safety. Listening requires a level of understanding that makes conversations more complex and, therefore, translates into a more developed skillset of interpersonal communication.

We must understand the natural human behavior tendencies to develop the professional relationships needed for psychological safety. Dr. Amy Edmonson refers to these characteristics as interpersonal risks. It is one's conscious or subconscious reaction to prevent looking stupid, incompetent, or disruptive [73]. This behavior is typically learned early when others around us begin to respond when we speak up. Think back to your earliest memory in the school of asking a question, and others laughed or criticized your question. Instantly, the feeling of inadequacy or incompetence created fear of taking that interpersonal risk again. This fear of inadequacy or incompetence can follow us into adulthood. In our professional careers, and even more so in health care, we set an expectation of ourselves to have the answer, execute the skill, or perform as if we have a natural ability. This expectation often prevents us from asking questions, seeking feedback, or being innovative for fear of how our colleagues will view us. When fear exists, we will remain silent when we should and need to speak.

As a leader, it is important to understand your behaviors in order to understand your 'staff's behavior. When we think of a lack of psychological safety, it is natural to associate this problem with lower-level staff. However, this problem can be experienced at the highest levels of an organization; thus, there is a need to have psychological safety created at the top and then cascaded throughout the organization. But how do you know if psychological safety exists in your organization? The most common method of measuring psychological safety is through a survey. Some regulatory requirements include conducting a patient safety culture survey. Several psychological safety surveys are available, which include questions about speaking up in the work setting, adequate disagreement resolution, a culture of learning from errors, and the ease of discussing these events [75].

2.4.4 Building the framework

Leaders build psychological safety by setting the stage, inviting participation, and responding productively. This framework is summarized as The 'Leader's Tool Kit and described by Amy C. Edmonson in her book, "The Fearless Organization" [73]. In her message, she offers practical guidance for organizations, healthcare institutions, and teams to succeed in the present technological environment, developing a culture where interpersonal interactions do not suppress, ridicule, silence, or intimidate any member. Leaders are role models by asking for help, using emotional intelligence, and discouraging behaviors leading to threatening psychological safety (**Figures 4** and **5**).

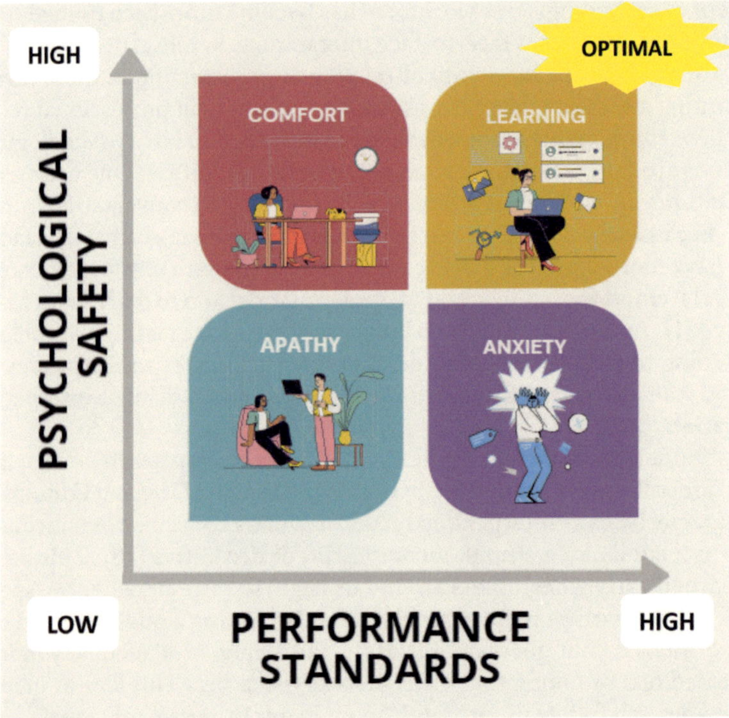

Figure 4.
Performance standards related to psychological safety. Comfort zone: Collegial and open, not challenged. A lack of initiative characterizes teamwork. Learning zone: Collaboration and a learning environment, high performance, excitement in getting involved in complex and innovative ideas. Apathy zone: Physical presence at work without deep involvement, self-preservation, or overexertion. Anxiety zone: Reluctance to offer new ideas, attempt new things, or ask for help. Mistrust. (based on [76]).

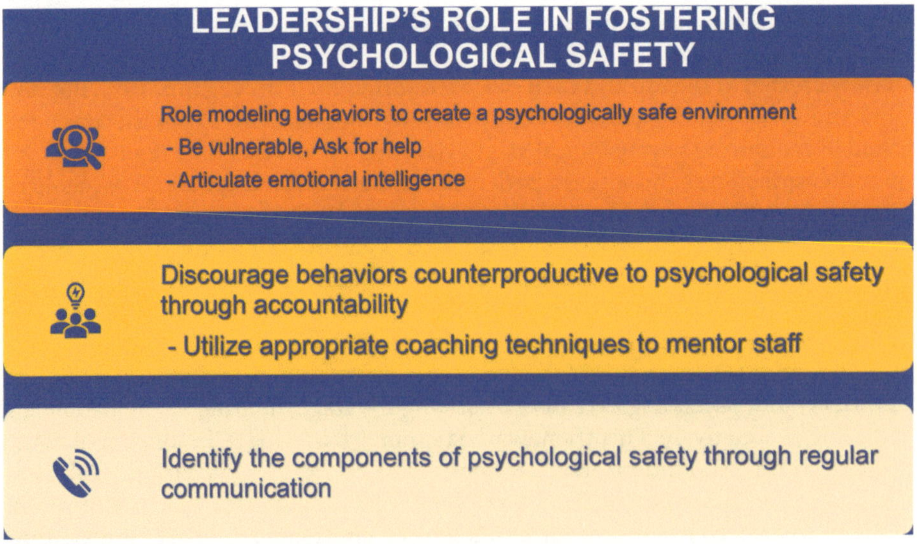

Figure 5.
'Leadership's role in enhancing psychological safety.

There are various ways to enhance psychological safety and enable a learning process in healthcare organizations, such as showing supportive leadership behaviors, building connections among team members, and using supportive organizational practices [77]. A different strategy emphasizes encouraging open dialog, scheduling leader presentations on speaking up, building a culture of trust, and making team members feel valued [78]. The common thread seems to be the importance of leadership involvement and their messaging while building an environment of trust and respect. Trust becomes 'visible' when team members willingly speak up and feel safe. However, building trust takes time and commitment from the leader. It is particularly challenging for teams to work remotely or for managers to lead staff in various locations. It can be done in a variety of ways, including scheduling and keeping one-on-one meetings, following through on commitments, promoting leadership transparency, and simply being available and present. If staff feel they have psychological safety, they will feel empowered to try new things, innovate and avoid 'workarounds' [73]. This can be seen when coaching quality improvement teams through their quality project work. Generally, project teams may not entertain the idea of becoming involved in quality improvement work without the autonomy to carry the project through to completion. Nor will they be inclined to produce innovative interventions if they believe they will not receive the buy-in or support required to implement. These concerns can be addressed early on by encouraging the selection of a project sponsor who will provide support throughout the project, remove barriers as needed, and help the team gain buy-in for their interventions [79]. Project sponsors are just one way to help reinforce a safe culture of creativity for project teams. Teams can also be encouraged to communicate often about their quality project work and incorporate change management techniques throughout the project lifecycle. Quality improvement efforts should not be considered additional work. Rather, once staff understands how to apply a structured problem-solving approach to improve outcomes, safety, and experience, the approach can be incorporated into daily work.

2.4.5 Balancing safety with accountability

a. How to respond to near misses: Near-miss events describe events where no actual harm comes to the patient. However, they represent an opportunity to improve patient safety and enhance communication with patients and families about disclosing medical errors [80]. An ideal transparent voluntary reporting system should enable structured reporting, collection and analysis of the data, and subsequent learning from these events when they are examined. A reporting system should be simple to access for reporting and have loop closure with the reporting individual to enhance satisfaction with the events that are addressed [81].

b. How to respond to never events: Preventable medical errors leading to a significant injury or death of patients are termed never events [82]. These events have been categorized into seven distinct groups. (**Table 4**). Because these events seriously affect patient safety and quality of care in hospitals, developing safety mechanisms to abolish their occurrence in the medical system has become a priority. Several adverse events registries have been designed to determine their frequency and include mandatory reporting, followed by methodology recommended by the Institute of Healthcare 'Improvement's Global Trigger Tool [83]. A systematic review specifically addressed the occurrence of the most common

Surgical or procedural	Surgery on the wrong part of the body Surgery or invasive procedure on the wrong patient Wrong surgical or invasive procedure on a patient Unintended retention of foreign object Intraoperative or immediately postoperative death
Product or device	Patient death or serious injury associated with contaminated devices or biologics Patient death or serious injury associated with the misuse or malfunction of a device Patient death or serious injury associated with intravascular air embolism
Patient protection	Discharge or release of a patient/resident of any age unable to make decisions Patient death or serious disability associated with patient elopement Patient suicide, attempted suicide while being cared for in a health care facility
Care management	Death or serious injury related to medication errors, unsafe administration of blood products, maternal death with labor or delivery in low-risk pregnancy Stage 3, 4, or unstageable pressure ulcers Falls leading to death or serious injury Failure to follow up or communicate laboratory, pathology, or radiology results
Environmental	Death or serious injury associated with electric shock, oxygen use, burn incurred from any source in the health care setting, use of restraints or bedrails
Radiological	Death or serious injury of a patient or staff related to the introduction of a metallic object into the MRI area
Criminal	Care is ordered by or provided by a physician, nurse, pharmacist, or other licensed healthcare provider impersonator.

Table 4.
Never events categories [82].

never events worldwide and by specialty, describing 60% of them as largely preventable [84], and the most common surgical ones include surgery on the wrong body part or patient and the wrong surgical procedure. Operating room checklists have become engrained in surgical practice to avoid these types of events [85].

One way to decrease the emotional impact of adverse events on healthcare providers is to provide the directly affected individual(s) with timely and adequate support, including peer-to-peer counseling, debriefing sessions, psychological consultations, or employee assistance programs. Healthcare organizations should foster a culture of care and compassion for their staff and a culture of safety and learning. The burnout risk in healthcare providers can be mitigated by acknowledging the human factors contributing to medical errors and promoting resilience and recovery among healthcare workers [26].

Ultimately, a strategic change in the healthcare system has been recommended to decrease, and ideally avoid, all never events. A systems approach to patient safety includes establishing and maintaining a safety culture, centralizing and coordinating oversite of patient safety, creating a standard set of safety metrics leading to meaningful outcomes, increasing funding for patient safety research and implementation science, addressing safety across a care continuum, supporting health care workforce, partnering with patients and families and ensuring that technology is safe and directed to optimize patient safety [86].

2.4.6 Navigating safety: evolution or revolution?

a. Safety 2.0

Safety 2.0 is a term that describes a new way of looking at safety management that emphasizes learning from what works well instead of what goes wrong. Safety 2.0 assumes that everyday performance variability enables the adaptations necessary to deal with changing conditions so things go right [87]. Safety 2.0 also acknowledges that humans are a resource essential for system flexibility and resilience rather than a cause of error and risk [88]. Safety 2.0 aims to understand how people and organizations achieve their goals under different situations and how to support and improve their performance [89]. Safety 2.0 differs from Safety 1.0, the traditional approach that focuses on accidents and tries to prevent bad outcomes by eliminating or minimizing hazards, errors, and failures.

b. Health 4.0

Health 4.0 is a concept that describes the use of Industry 4.0 technologies, such as artificial intelligence, big data, cloud computing, the internet of things, and blockchain, in the health care sector (**Table 5**) [90]. Health 4.0 has the goal of improving the quality, accessibility, efficiency, and personalization of healthcare services, as well as of empowering patients and healthcare professionals [91].

The relationship between Health 4.0 and safety is a crucial and complex issue, as it involves both possible advantages and challenges. On the one hand, Health 4.0 can improve the safety of patients and health care workers by facilitating better diagnosis, treatment, monitoring, and prevention of diseases and injuries and by minimizing human errors, waste, and costs [91]. On the other hand, Health 4.0 can also create new risks and threats to safety, such as cyberattacks, data breaches, ethical dilemmas, legal liabilities, and social inequalities [93].

Stage	Description
Health 1.0	This was the traditional healthcare system, which mainly reacted to health problems and provided care in hospitals and clinics. The emphasis was on curing diseases rather than preventing them, and there was little use of technology.
Health 2.0	In this stage, electronic health records and health information exchanges were introduced, and digital data started to be used, but still within the limits of the traditional healthcare model.
Health 3.0	In this stage, technology became more integrated into patient care, with a focus on personalized medicine and patient involvement. Technologies such as telemedicine, mobile health apps, and wearable devices became more common, allowing for more data-driven and patient-focused care.
Health 4.0	Based on the previous stages, Health 4.0 is marked by a fully integrated, digital healthcare system. It uses advanced technologies like AI, big data analytics, and the Internet of Things to provide proactive, predictive, and personalized healthcare services. The aim is to achieve a smooth patient experience and improved health outcomes through the combination of cyber and physical systems.

Table 5.
Steps towards a more interconnected, efficient, and patient-focused healthcare system, from health 1.0 to 4.0. [92].

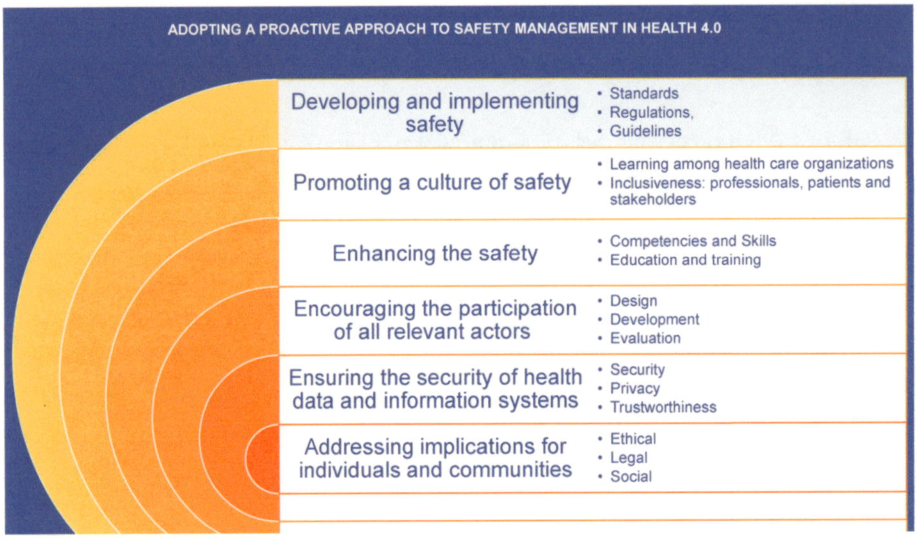

Figure 6.
Adopting a Proactive Approach to Safety Management in Health 4-0. This figure illustrates the multifaceted strategy for enhancing safety in healthcare by promoting a culture of safety, encouraging inclusive participation, ensuring data security, and addressing community implications through standards, regulations, and education.

c. Virtual workers

Virtual work enables employees to do their work from a different location, such as home or a remote center, using technology to connect and cooperate with their co-workers and customers [94]. Virtual work can provide enhanced safety, flexibility, productivity, and innovation advantages (**Figure 6**) [95].

Virtual healthcare employees must feel included for their well-being, engagement, and performance. Some ways to achieve these goals are: The use of various communication tools, such as video calls, chat apps, and social media, to create a sense of connection and belonging among remote workers [96]. Have regular check-ins with remote workers, individually and as a team, to give feedback, support, and recognition [96]. Include remote workers in decision-making and goal-setting processes, enabling them to make choices and take initiative [97, 98]. Acknowledge and appreciate each remote 'worker's contribution publicly and privately and provide opportunities for learning and growth [97].

Support remote workers in sharing their values, interests, and personal stories and build workplace friendships through virtual social events and activities [97]. Be aware of time zones and cultural differences when scheduling meetings and events and ensure remote workers can access information and resources equally [99]. A graphic representation of the evaluation and implementation of virtual work is described in (**Figure** 7).

3. Conclusion

In conclusion, this chapter has provided an overview of the current trends and challenges in the healthcare sector and how they affect patients' and providers' safety and well-being. It has also discussed the components of high-reliability organizations

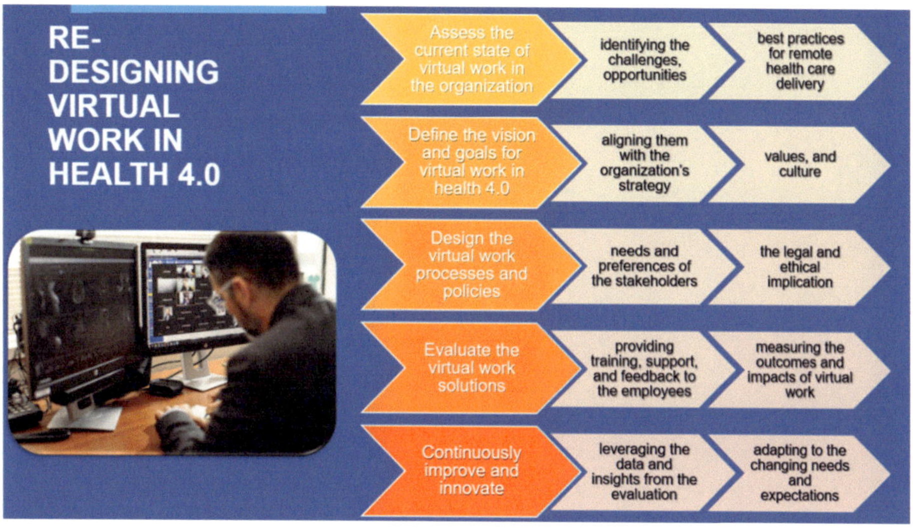

Figure 7.
Re-designing Virtual Work in Health 4.0 - This figure outlines a comprehensive approach to re-evaluating and enhancing virtual work within healthcare settings. It emphasizes the importance of assessing the current state, defining clear vision and goals, designing effective work processes and policies, evaluating virtual work solutions, and fostering continuous improvement and innovation.

and how they can create a culture of safety and human connection in the face of uncertainty and complexity. Furthermore, it has explored the concept of Safety 2.0, which emphasizes learning from what works well instead of what goes wrong, the relationship between Health 4.0 and safety, and the challenges and opportunities of virtual work. Lastly, it has explained the importance of unpretentious leadership and trust in building psychological safety, which is the feeling of speaking up without fear of negative consequences, and the best practices for onboarding new employees and setting expectations for safety behaviors.

This chapter aims to provide valuable insights and recommendations for healthcare leaders, managers, and workers who want to improve the safety and quality of their services and their own mental and emotional health. However, it is essential to acknowledge that there is no one-size-fits-all solution for achieving these goals and that each organization and individual needs to adapt and thrive in the dynamic and demanding healthcare environment. Therefore, we encourage readers to reflect on the concepts and ideas presented in this chapter, apply them in their contexts and situations, and seek feedback and learn from others.

Notes/thanks/other declarations

We want to thank our mentors, colleagues, and learners who inspired us to seek ways to improve our current medical system. Most importantly, we are grateful to our patients, from whom we have learned how to become better healthcare professionals and best serve their needs. Without this collaboration, this chapter would have been incomplete

Author details

Pablo Moreno Franco[1], LaRissa Adams[1], Sandy C. Booth[1] and Grace M. Arteaga[2*]

1 Mayo Clinic, Florida, USA

2 Mayo Clinic Rochester, Minnesota, USA

*Address all correspondence to: arteaga.grace@mayo.edu

IntechOpen

© 2024 The Author(s). Licensee IntechOpen. This chapter is distributed under the terms of the Creative Commons Attribution License (http://creativecommons.org/licenses/by/3.0), which permits unrestricted use, distribution, and reproduction in any medium, provided the original work is properly cited.

References

[1] Chen C et al. The times they are a-Changin' - healthcare 4.0 is coming! Journal of Medical Systems. 2019;**44**(2):40. DOI: 10.1007/s10916-019-1513-0

[2] Domínguez-Miranda SA, Rodríguez-Aguilar R. Health 4.0, prevention, and health promotion in companies: A systematic literature review. In: Marmolejo-Saucedo JA, Rodríguez-Aguilar R, Vasant P, Litvinchev I, Retana-Blanco BM, editors. Computer Science and Engineering in Health Services. COMPSE 2022. Cham: Springer; 2024. DOI: 10.1007/978-3-031-34750-4_13

[3] Kang J, Cho YJ, Choi S. State anxiety, uncertainty in illness, and needs of family members of critically ill patients and their experiences with family-centered multidisciplinary rounds: A mixed model study. PLoS One. 2020;**15**(6):e0234296. DOI: 10.1371/journal.pone.0234296

[4] Verhaeghe S, Defloor T, Grypdonck M. Stress and coping among families of patients with traumatic brain injury: A review of the literature. Journal of Clinical Nursing. 2005;**14**(8):1004-1012. DOI: 10.1111/j.1365-2702.2005.01126.x

[5] Liu T et al. Impact of COVID-19 infection experience on mental health status of intensive care unit patients' family members: A real-world study. QJM. 2023;**116**(11):903-910. DOI: 10.1093/qjmed/hcad184

[6] Kynoch K et al. The effectiveness of interventions to meet family needs of critically ill patients in an adult intensive care unit: A systematic review update. JBI Database of Systematic Reviews and Implementation Reports. 2016;**14**(3):181-234. DOI: 10.11124/JBISRIR-2016-2477

[7] Park M et al. Patient- and family-centered care interventions for improving the quality of health care: A review of systematic reviews. International Journal of Nursing Studies. 2018;**87**:69-83. DOI: 10.1016/j.ijnurstu.2018.07.006

[8] Goldfarb M, Bibas L, Burns K. Patient and family engagement in Care in the Cardiac Intensive Care Unit. The Canadian Journal of Cardiology. 2020;**36**(7):1032-1040. DOI: 10.1016/j.cjca.2020.03.037

[9] Farrier CE, Stelfox HT, Fiest KM. In the pursuit of partnership: Patient and family engagement in critical care medicine. Current Opinion in Critical Care. 2019;**25**(5):505-510. DOI: 10.1097/MCC.0000000000000643

[10] Kean L, Milner KA. Implementation of open visitation in an adult intensive care unit: An evidence-based practice quality improvement project. Critical Care Nurse. 2020;**40**(2):76-79. DOI: 10.4037/ccn2020661

[11] Silvera GA, Clark JR. Women at the helm: Chief executive officer gender and patient experience in the hospital industry. Health Care Management Review. 2021;**46**(3):206-216. DOI: 10.1097/HMR.0000000000000252

[12] Dragoi L, Munshi L, Herridge M. Visitation policies in the ICU and the importance of family presence at the bedside. Intensive Care Medicine. 2022;**48**(12):1790-1792. DOI: 10.1007/s00134-022-06848-1

[13] Manary MP et al. The patient experience and health outcomes.

The New England Journal of Medicine. 2013;**368**(3):201-203. DOI: 10.1056/NEJMp1211775

[14] Doyle C, Lennox L, Bell D. A systematic review of evidence on the links between patient experience and clinical safety and effectiveness. BMJ Open. 2013;**3**(1). DOI: 10.1136/bmjopen-2012-001570

[15] Martin D. Physical environment impacts patient experience. Health Facilities Management. 2016;**29**(5):39

[16] Gabay G. Patient self-worth and communication barriers to Trust of Israeli Patients in acute-care physicians at public general hospitals. Qualitative Health Research. 2019;**29**(13):1954-1966. DOI: 10.1177/1049732319844999

[17] Clark CC. Trust in medicine. The Journal of Medicine and Philosophy. 2002;**27**(1):11-29. DOI: 10.1076/jmep.27.1.11.2975

[18] Abid MH et al. Patient engagement and patient safety: Are we missing the patient in the Center? Cureus. 2020;**12**(2):e7048. DOI: 10.7759/cureus.7048

[19] Dzakula A, Relic D. Health workforce shortage - doing the right things or doing things right? Croatian Medical Journal. 2022;**63**(2):107-109. DOI: 10.3325/cmj.2022.63.107

[20] Endacott R et al. The organisation of nurse staffing in intensive care units: A qualitative study. Journal of Nursing Management. 2022;**30**(5):1283-1294. DOI: 10.1111/jonm.13611

[21] Hooiveld J. How staffing shortages affect patient safety in healthcare and nursing. In: Patient Safety. Symplr company; 2024. Available from: https://www.patientsafety.com/en/blog/staffing-shortages-affects-patient-safety

[22] Roche E et al. Learning lessons from the paediatric critical care response to the SARS-CoV-2 pandemic in England and Wales: A qualitative study. Archives of Disease in Childhood. 2022;**107**(3):e6. DOI: 10.1136/archdischild-2020-320662

[23] Aiken LH et al. Hospital nurse staffing and patient mortality, nurse burnout, and job dissatisfaction. JAMA. 2002;**288**(16):1987-1993. DOI: 10.1001/jama.288.16.1987

[24] Rosenberg K. RN shortages negatively impact patient safety. The American Journal of Nursing. 2019;**119**(3):51. DOI: 10.1097/01.NAJ.0000554040.98991.23

[25] Hall LH et al. Healthcare staff well-being, burnout, and patient safety: A systematic review. PLoS One. 2016;**11**(7):e0159015. DOI: 10.1371/journal.pone.0159015

[26] Yates SW. Physician stress and burnout. The American Journal of Medicine. 2020;**133**(2):160-164. DOI: 10.1016/j.amjmed.2019.08.034

[27] Salyers MP et al. The relationship between professional burnout and quality and safety in healthcare: A meta-analysis. Journal of General Internal Medicine. 2017;**32**(4):475-482. DOI: 10.1007/s11606-016-3886-9

[28] Tawfik DS et al. Physician burnout, well-being, and work unit safety grades in relationship to reported medical errors. Mayo Clinic Proceedings. 2018;**93**(11):1571-1580. DOI: 10.1016/j.mayocp.2018.05.014

[29] West CP et al. Association of perceived medical errors with resident distress and empathy: A prospective longitudinal study. JAMA. 2006;**296**(9):1071-1078. DOI: 10.1001/jama.296.9.1071

[30] Buchbinder M, Berlinger N, Jenkins TM. Protecting practitioners in stressed systems: Translational bioethics and the COVID-19 pandemic. Perspectives in Biology and Medicine. 2022;**65**(4):637-645. DOI: 10.1353/pbm.2022.0055

[31] Buchbinder M, Jenkins T. Burnout in critical care: Time for moving upstream. Annals of the American Thoracic Society. 2022;**19**(9):1443-1445. DOI: 10.1513/AnnalsATS.202202-111IP

[32] Seaman JB, Cohen TR, White DB. Reducing the stress on clinicians working in the ICU. JAMA. 2018;**320**(19):1981-1982. DOI: 10.1001/jama.2018.14285

[33] Jordan SR, Connors SC, Mastalerz KA. Frontline healthcare workers' perspectives on interprofessional teamwork during COVID-19. Journal of Interprofessional Education & Practice. 2022;**29**:100550. DOI: 10.1016/j.xjep.2022.100550

[34] Hopkins A. A Practical Guide to Becoming a High Reliability Organization. High Reliability Organizations (HRO). Australian Institute of Health & Safety (AIHS); 2021 Available from: https://www.aihs.org.au/common/Uploaded%20files/About-us/Policy/A-Practical-Guide-to-becoming-a-High-Reliability-Organisation-Andrew-Hopkins.pdf

[35] Grazman D. The Pursuit of Zero Harm Introducing High Reliability Concepts to Community Health Centers. Joint Commission Center for Transforming Healthcare. The Joint Commission; 2019 Available from: https://www.jointcommission.org/-/media/tjc/documents/accred-and-cert/ahc/the_pursuit_of_zero_harm.pdf?db=web&hash=1DAD6BF19C36DAFEB153364D931602C0

[36] Ameze O, Odiase K. Organizational safety culture transformation through coaching. International Journal of Innovative Research & Development. 2022;**11**(10):8-14. DOI: 10.24940/ijird/2022/v11/i10/OCT22001

[37] Card AJ. Patient safety 2.0: Slaying dragons, not just investigating them. Journal of Patient Safety. 2023;**19**(6):394-395. DOI: 10.1097/PTS.0000000000001140

[38] Costa F et al. How to foster sustainable continuous improvement: A cause-effect relations map of lean soft practices. Operations Research Perspectives. 2019;**6**:100091. DOI: 10.1016/j.orp.2018.100091

[39] Veazie S, Peterson K, Bourne D. In: W.D.D.o.V.A. (US), editor. Evidence Brief: Implementation of High Reliability Organization Principles. Washington (DC), USA: Department of Veterans Affairs (US); 2019

[40] Sutcliffe KM. High reliability organizations (HROs). Best Practice & Research. Clinical Anaesthesiology. 2011;**25**(2):133-144. DOI: 10.1016/j.bpa.2011.03.001

[41] Abrams K, Shudes C, Shah U. Virtual health: Extending the human touch in care delivery. Deloitte; 2019 Available from: https://www2.deloitte.com/content/dam/Deloitte/us/Documents/life-sciences-health-care/us-lshc-virtual-health-care-physcian-adoption.pdf

[42] Cooley L. Fostering human connection in the Covid-19 virtual health care realm. The New England Journal of Medicine Catalyst. 20 May 2020:1-6. DOI: 10.1056/CAT.20.0166

[43] Smith W. Balancing Digital Innovation and Human Connection: The Critical Role of Personal Interaction in

Healthcare. HealthSnap. HealthSnap; 2024 Available from: https://healthsnap.io/balancing-digital-innovation-and-human-connection-the-critical-role-of-personal-interaction-in-healthcare/

[44] Bojic Z. High Reliability Organizations (HROs). SYSTEMICO Systems Thinking. Process Excellence. Sustainable Results. SYSTEMICO; 2015 [cited 2024 March 8]; Available from: https://www.systemico.ca/high-reliability-organizations-hros/

[45] Terry C, Cain J. The emerging issue of digital empathy. American Journal of Pharmaceutical Education. 2016;**80**(4):58. DOI: 10.5688/ajpe80458

[46] Radin J, Bordeaux C, Schwartz J. Closing the Employability Skills Gap: The Answer Is Simpler than you May Think; 2020. Available from: https://www2.deloitte.com/us/en/insights/focus/technology-and-the-future-of-work/closing-the-employability-skills-gap.html

[47] Morrison-Smith S, Ruiz J. Challenges and barriers in virtual teams: A literature review. Sn. Applied Sciences. 2020;**2**(6):1096. DOI: 10.1007/s42452-020-2801-5

[48] Adams N, Allen R, Ojukwu E. Workplace Redesign: Current Trends, Challenges, and Opportunities. ILR CAHRS. Cornell University; 2019. Available from: https://est05.esalestrack.com/eSalesTrack/Content/Content.ashx?file=89d39838-fd4a-4dcc-b3f2-cdb4fc61d66e.pdf

[49] Glass G. Navigating The Onboarding Process For A Remote Workforce. Forbes Leadership. Forbes.com; 2022. Available from: https://www.forbes.com/sites/forbeshumanresourcescouncil/2022/02/15/navigating-the-onboarding-process-for-a-remote-workforce/?sh=f4f64b130a38

[50] Zucker R. How to Re-Onboard Employees Who Started Remotely. Harvard Business Review. Harvard Business Publisher; 2021. Available from: https://hbr.org/2021/06/how-to-re-onboard-employees-who-started-remotely

[51] Leadership, C.f.C. Better Culture Starts with Better Conversations. Center for creative Leadership. Center for Creative Leadership; 2023. Available from: https://www.ccl.org/articles/white-papers/better-culture-starts-with-better-conversations/

[52] Commission, TJ Sentinel Event Data 2022 Annual Review; 2023. Available from: https://www.jointcommission.org/-/media/tjc/documents/resources/patient-safety-topics/sentinel-event/03162023_sentinel-event-_annual-review_final.pdf

[53] Starmer AJ et al. Improving handoffs in the perioperative environment: A conceptual framework of key theories, system factors, methods, and Core interventions to ensure success. Joint Commission Journal on Quality and Patient Safety. 2023;**49**(8):384-393. DOI: 10.1016/j.jcjq.2023.06.006

[54] BC, S. Safety Huddles. SafeCare BC; 2024. Available from: https://safecarebc.ca/resources/huddles/

[55] Wagner C, Theel A, Handel S. Safety Huddles. Guide to Safety Huddles. A Culture of Safety: Bringing Board Members, Executive Leaders, and Staff Together. Washington State Hospital Association; 2015. Available from: https://www.wsha.org/wp-content/uploads/Worker-Safety_SafetyHuddleToolkit_3_27_15.pdf

[56] Stahl S. The Evolution of Aviation Safety. Aero Crew News; 2016. Available from: https://aerocrewnews.com/

education-2/safetywx/safety-matters/the-evolution-of-aviation-safety/

[57] Aerosystems, H. The History of Aviation Safety. HRD; 2018 Available from: https://www.hrd-aerosystems.com/blog/history-of-aviation-safety/

[58] Administration FA. Out Front on Airline Safety: Two Decades of Continuous Evolution. United States Department of Transportation; 2018. Available from: https://www.faa.gov/newsroom/out-front-airline-safety-two-decades-continuous-evolution

[59] Shaikh U. Improving Patient Safety and Team Communication through Daily Huddles. Patient Safety. Agency for Healthcare Research and Quality (AHRQ); 2020. Available from: https://psnet.ahrq.gov/primer/improving-patient-safety-and-team-communication-through-daily-huddles

[60] CommissionCE. Safety Huddles: Implementation Guide. Safety Huddles. National Library of Australia Cataloguing-in Publication; 2017. Available from: https://www.cec.health.nsw.gov.au/improve-quality/teamwork-culture-pcc/safety-fundamentals/for-teams/safety-huddles

[61] Franklin BJ et al. Impact of multidisciplinary team huddles on patient safety: A systematic review and proposed taxonomy. BMJ Quality and Safety. 2020;**29**(10):1-2. DOI: 10.1136/bmjqs-2019-009911

[62] Rakover J. 5 Tips for Better Huddles. Patient Safety: Handoffs In Healthcare. Institute for Healthcare Improvement (IHI); 2018. Available from: https://www.ihi.org/insights/5-tips-better-huddles

[63] Within3. How Huddles in Healthcare can Improve the Patient Experience. Within3; 2022. Available from: https://within3.com/blog/huddles-in-healthcare

[64] Health, R.R.C.o.P.a.C. Safety Huddles – Rules & Standardised Script. SAFE Toolkit Module 3 - From Reaction to Anticipation (2018). Available from: https://www.rcpch.ac.uk/sites/default/files/2018-04/safe_5c_-_gosh_safety_huddle_script.pdf

[65] Commission, CE. Safety Huddles: Information for Clinicians & Health Professionals. Clinical Excellence Commission NSW Government. New South Wales, Australia: Safety Huddles Info for Clinicians; 22 April 2024. Available from: (nsw.gov.au)

[66] Partners PH. How to Conduct Effective Safety Huddle. Safety Huddles Whitepaper. Performance Health Partners; 2023. Available from: https://www.performancehealthus.com/blog/how-to-conduct-effective-safety-huddles

[67] Goldenhar LM et al. Huddling for high reliability and situation awareness. BMJ Quality and Safety. 2013;**22**(11):899-906. DOI: 10.1136/bmjqs-2012-001467

[68] Lamming L et al. Fidelity and the impact of patient safety huddles on teamwork and safety culture: An evaluation of the huddle up for safer healthcare (HUSH) project. BMC Health Services Research. 2021;**21**(1):1038. DOI: 10.1186/s12913-021-07080-1

[69] Wang Y, Liu J, Zhu Y. Humble leadership, psychological safety, knowledge sharing, and follower creativity: A cross-level investigation. Frontiers in Psychology. 2018;**9**:1727. DOI: 10.3389/fpsyg.2018.01727

[70] Carmeli A, Reiter-Palmon R, Ziv E. Inclusive leadership and employee involvement in creative tasks in the workplace: The mediating role of psychological safety. Creativity Research Journal. 2010;**22**(3):250-260. Online. DOI: 10.1080/10400419.2010.504654

[71] Rego A, Melo AI, Bluhm DJ, et al. Leader-expressed humility predicting team psychological safety: A personality dynamics lens. Journal of Business Ethics. 2021;**174**:669-686. DOI: 10.1007/s10551-020-04622-1

[72] Legood A, van der Werff L, Den Hartog D. A meta-analysis of the role of trust in the leadership-performance relationship. European Journal of Work and Organizational Psychology. 2021;**1**(30):1-22. DOI: 10.1080/1359432X.2020.1819241

[73] Edmonson AC. In: School HB, editor. The Fearless Organization. New Jersey USA: John Wiley & Son; 2018

[74] Thomas L, Rodziewicz BH, John E. Hipskind. Medical Error Reduction and Prevention. StatPearls [Internet]; 2023. Available from: https://www.ncbi.nlm.nih.gov/books/NBK499956/

[75] Adair KC et al. The psychological safety scale of the safety, communication, operational, reliability, and engagement (SCORE) survey: A brief, diagnostic, and actionable metric for the ability to speak up in healthcare settings. Journal of Patient Safety. 2022;**18**(6):513-520. DOI: 10.1097/PTS.0000000000001048

[76] Edmonson A. How Psychological Safety Relates to Performance Standards. Psychological Safety. Amyedmonson.com; 2022. Available from: https://amycedmondson.com/psychological-safety-%E2%89%A0-anything-goes/

[77] Newman A, Donohue R, Eva N. Psychological safety: A systematic review of the literature. Human Resource Management Review. 2017;**27**:521-535. DOI: 10.1016/j.hrmr.2017.01.001

[78] Murray JS, Kelly S, Hanover C. Promoting psychological safety in healthcare organizations. Military Medicine. 2022;**187**(7-8):808-810. DOI: 10.1093/milmed/usac041

[79] Banchs RJ, Pop MR. The Quality Improvement Challenge: A Practical Guide for Physicians. First ed. Oxford, UK: Wiley-Blackwell; 2021

[80] Crane S, Sloane PD, Elder NC, Cohen LW, Laughtenschlager N, Zimmerman S. Implementing near-miss reporting and improvement tracking in primary care practices: Lessons learned. Advances in Patient Safety and Medical Liability. Agency for Healthcare Research and Quality (ahrq.gov). 2017. Available from: https://www.ahrq.gov/patient-safety/reports/liability/crane.html

[81] Mahmoud HA et al. Barriers and facilitators to improving patient safety learning systems: A systematic review of qualitative studies and meta-synthesis. BMJ Open Quality. 2023;**12**(2). DOI: 10.1136/bmjoq-2022-002134

[82] Agency for Healthcare Research and Quality. Never Events. Patient Safety 101. Agency for Heathcare Research and Quality; 2019. Available from: https://psnet.ahrq.gov/primer/never-events

[83] Griffin FA, Resar RK. IHI Global Trigger Tool for Measuring Adverse Events (White Paper). Improvement Areas. Institute for Healthcare Improvement; 2009. Available from: https://www.ihi.org/resources/white-papers/ihi-global-trigger-tool-measuring-adverse-events

[84] Bowman CL, De Gorter R, Zaslow J, Fortier JH, Garber G. Identifying a list of healthcare 'never events' to effect system change: A systematic review and narrative synthesis. BMJ Open Quality. 2023;**12**(2):e002264. DOI: 10.1136/bmjoq-2023-002264. PMID: 37364940; PMCID: PMC10314656

[85] Hepner DL et al. Operating room crisis checklists and emergency manuals.

Anesthesiology. 2017;**127**(2):384-392. DOI: 10.1097/ALN.0000000000001731

[86] Lark ME, Kirkpatrick K, Chung KC. Patient safety movement: History and future directions. The Journal of Hand Surgery. 2018;**43**(2):174-178. DOI: 10.1016/j.jhsa.2017.11.006

[87] Hollnagel E, Wears RL, Braithwaite J. From Safety-I to Safety-II: A White Paper. Published simultaneously by the University of Southern Denmark, University of Florida, USA, and Macquarie University, Australia; 2015. Available from: https://www.england.nhs.uk/signuptosafety/wp-content/uploads/sites/16/2015/10/safety-1-safety-2-whte-papr.pdf

[88] Company TPS. The Safety-II Approach: Learning from What Goes Right. Patient Safety. The Patient Safety Company: a symplr company; 2024. Available from: https://www.patientsafety.com/en/blog/safety-2-versus-safety-1

[89] Safety4Sea. Safety I vs Safety II: An overview. Safety. 2018; Available from: https://safety4sea.com/cm-safety-i-vs-safety-ii-an-overview/

[90] Polak-Sopinska A, Wisniewski Z, Walaszczyk A, Maczewska A, Sopinski P. Impact of industry 4.0 on occupational health and safety. In: International Conference on Applied Human Factors and Ergonomics. Springer Link; 2019. Available from: https://link.springer.com/chapter/10.1007/978-3-030-20494-5_4

[91] Musarat, M.A., Salah Alaloul, W., Irfan, I., Sreenivasan, P., Rabbani, M.B.A. Health and Safety Improvement through Industrial Revolution 4.0: Malaysian Construction Industry Case. Sustainability (2022); MDPI; Available from: https://www.mdpi.com/2071-1050/15/1/201#

[92] Li J, Carayon P. Health care 4.0: A vision for smart and connected health care. IISE transactions on healthcare. Systems Engineering. 2021;**11**:1-14. DOI: 10.1080/24725579.2021.1884627

[93] Association, A.M. Advancing Health Care AI Through Ethics, Evidence and Equity. Artificial Intelligence. American Medical Association; 2018. Available from: https://www.ama-assn.org/practice-management/digital/advancing-health-care-ai-through-ethics-evidence-and-equity

[94] M., B. Implementing And Enabling A Virtual Workforce. Leadership. Forbes; 2020. Available from: https://www.forbes.com/sites/forbescoachescouncil/2020/05/05/implementing-and-enabling-a-virtual-workforce/?sh=7d66949d7575

[95] Healthineers S. The Case for Remote Work in Health Care. Harvard Business Review. Harvard Business Review; 2020. Available from: https://hbr.org/sponsored/2020/09/the-case-for-remote-work-in-health-care

[96] Panel E. 15 Ways To Ensure Remote Workers Feel Included In Company Culture. Forbes Human Resources Council. Forbes; 2021. Available from: https://www.forbes.com/sites/forbeshumanresourcescouncil/2021/04/02/15-ways-to-ensure-remote-workers-feel-included-in-company-culture/?sh=46be18881c52

[97] Ross H. How to Make Remote Employees Feel Included and Engaged (12 Best Practices). Management. Fellow; 2021. Available from: https://fellow.app/blog/management/how-to-make-remote-employees-feel-included-and-engaged-best-practices/

[98] Booth RG, Strudwick G. Preparing nursing for the virtual care realities of a post-pandemic future.

Nursing Leadership (Toronto, Ont.). 2021;**34**(4):86-96. DOI: 10.12927/cjnl.2021.26685

[99] Panel E. 12 Ways To Help Remote Workers Feel Included In Company Culture. Leadership. Forbes; 2020. Available from: https://www.forbes.com/sites/forbeshumanresourcescouncil/2020/01/07/12-ways-to-help-remote-workers-feel-included-in-company-culture/?sh=3cbdddb45979

Chapter 3

Restructuring the Informed Consent to Treatment to Reduce Narratives of Regret

An Goldbauer

Abstract

Informed consent [IC] is a verbal agreement or standardized legalese with medical jargon few understand. Spending little time with the patient to meet numbers and generate profit in fulfilling the basic minimum criteria may result in patients experiencing regret. IC is more about reducing legal liability for the provider and less costly options for the insurance company as opposed to what the patient needs to know about their provider's training with gender-affirming care and surgery [GACS]. The patient must understand the risks when consenting to GACS that may result in regret months or years later. World Professional Association for Transgender Health [WPATH], standards of care, version 8 [SOC8], recommends GACS providers continue with their training and education but does not conduct medical or surgical oversight. Collaboration and coordinated care among providers and staff are sometimes lacking. Patients reported that their providers abandoned them post surgery. This author recommends restructuring the informed consent to include the physician/surgeon's training and the volume of cases treated, including critical providers involved with the patient's mental and medical care, and disclosing surgical complications and mortality risk. The author will address the need for accreditation.

Keywords: transgender care, informed consent, narratives of regret, gender-affirming care, formal training

1. Introduction

The average patient's expectation that surgeons must have training before embarking on gender-affirming surgery [GAS] is misleading. There are no formal guidelines or stipulations as there are with other types of surgeries. In general, surgeons typically do not disclose the volumes of GAS cases [1, 2].

WPATH serves as an International, multidisciplinary professional association whose global members range from various clinical and anthropological backgrounds who establish ethical guidelines, and high standards of care, develop best practices and policies for physicians treating and seeing individuals for gender-affirming care and surgery [GACS] using the Delphi Technique, a scientific evidence-based process. WPATH members range from nurses, physician assistants, medical doctors, surgeons, and therapists to psychiatrists, among many others in the medical and mental health field. WPATH SOC8 reminds professionals serving the transgender and gender-diverse [TGD] population that the gold standard of care is more about delivering expert, safe, compassionate care and offering more resources to access care. WPATH offers mentoring and certification [3].

In 2018, a WPATH open letter from transgender individuals with lived experience called for oversight, intervention, transparency, and the need for accreditation to reduce harm to the community by WPATH surgeons capitalizing on the trans population to gain experience. Some pursuing legal action for poor surgical outcomes and abandonment. They further called for accountability when surgeons need to be held to a higher standard since they are WPATH members [4, 5].

2. Informed consent and the need for transparency

Parents seeking guidance on behalf of their child or young adolescent need more advice and support, when providers assume to treat the child without thoroughly evaluating the history for mental health comorbidities or whether the child has been under a tremendous amount of peer pressure or social isolation. Parents report they often cannot connect with a clinician who does not recommend puberty blockers or hormone replacement therapy [HRT] [6]. American Medical Association [AMA], the organization for the Code of Medical Ethics and the first to nationally develop IC, defines it as necessary for medical and surgical treatments and to ensure that patients receive information and can ask questions about the risks and benefits before making an informed decision. The physician assesses if the patient can comprehend the diagnosis, the recommendations for treatment, benefits, risks, and alternatives. It is an ethical and legal obligation for all providers to cover the IC with the patient, and many states use the required standard based on what a typical patient needs to know and have been given options and alternatives [7, 8].

Authors studying risk in coronary artery bypass procedure [CABP] disclaim that the burden is placed upon patients to seek information about a surgeon's or physician's expertise and experience. Still, short of asking directly for this information, some providers aren't openly transparent. When the patient does not know to ask, they will not know that the provider does not have the training or performed enough surgical volumes. Having this information ahead of time may help the patient decide whether or not they want the surgeon to perform surgery. Without this knowledge, the patient is taking a risk when the surgeon's experience is not readily transparent. The authors recommend report card grading would raise transparency and be helpful to patients. Outcomes are predictable, hinging on the surgeon's experience, and since some surgeries are riskier than others adding the risk information would be material to the IC. The IC cannot be considered informed when material risk information is withheld. Previously this type of information would have been kept internally, but with time the public is pressuring providers, institutions, government, and insurance companies to disclose material risks [9].

Angie's List, healthgrades and consumer reports include physician/surgeon and hospital ratings. Some medical doctors critique this service as insufficient because it cannot be compared to those skilled in a trade, and the reviews are minimal and none of the reviews include experience, training or medical and surgical volumes, according to USA Today [10].

Patients could obtain information about malpractice suits against physicians through the Federation of State Medical Boards [FSMB], but this is a voluntary credentialing service that charges members for a fixed fee. It is not approved as a credentialing service by Joint Commission, National Committee for Quality Assurance [NCQA], or Det Norske Veritas [DNV] [11].

In a study examining medical errors and full disclosure, not all physicians were comfortable, worried about alienating patients, feared being sued and ending up in malpractice. Historically hospitals would deny any wrongdoing. Physicians were comfortable covering adverse events, but not talking about errors. Patients were less apt to file a lawsuit when the physician fully disclosed the error with an apology. Not all states disclose malpractice information. Currently, there are eight states that prohibit admission of error in court [12].

In a Georgetown law review, some states determined that information about a provider's credentials or experience with a given procedure may need to be disclosed on the IC through Artificial Intelligence [AI], mainly to reduce increased risks of injuries. While the law review did not address gender-affirming surgery, it did address other types of surgeries where a patient's IC in the section on Substitute Physicians, did not mention that a non-doctor would perform a portion of their surgery. In some of these events, patients experienced complications and sued. In the same section on Substitute Physicians, patients were not necessarily informed when surgeons were part of a team since deciding who would operate would not occur up until right before surgery. This practice is referred to as Ghost surgery or overlapping surgery when another surgeon steps in to perform part of the surgery [13].

In a Florida State Law Review, critics argue that as a nation, we over-treat versus under-treat to capitalize on gains when some unnecessary treatments harm the patient. The critics establish that fraud occurs based on failure to show that there was a medical necessity, rendering the IC inadequate. The information would afford a patient a better outcome, but some clinicians do not agree that they would make better clinical decisions. Some state that this is a false belief rather than checking the patient's level of understanding. The IC is regarded as a worthless document that disregards a number of discussions at the discretion of the physicians/surgeons. When things go wrong, or there are complications that were never covered in the IC, third-party payers are usually left out. If the False Claims Act [FCA] were involved, then claims filed for reimbursement could be denied when the physician/surgeon failed to provide the promised services, did not discuss complications with the patient, provided unnecessary service/treatment, or abandoned the patient. The Law Review points out that when the surgeon claims that care was medically necessary when it was not, then they have essentially committed fraud. The review points out that if the regulatory body linked the third-party payer, the third-party payer could deny payment for services [14].

Most patients would opt differently if the level of the surgeon's or physician's expertise with the volume of cases treated is public. Johns Hopkins in 2016 added a web page titled *Volume Pledge* to list patient safety for public transparency. Mortality with some surgeries is highest when surgeons have performed one or two surgeries and lowest when surgeons have performed high number of same surgeries [15, 16].

3. AI, collaboration, and the informed consent

The algorithm to treat or not to treat hinges on how experienced the provider is in treating individuals seeking medical/surgical treatments. In the first paragraph of the introduction, the authors refer to Walsh study on AIs ability to predict suicidal ideation and attempts based on patients health records but further in the section of the Pitfalls of AI, algorithms involve a profile of a patient with a specific ethnicity that may not apply to a patient whose ethnicity is different [17]. In the Georgetown Law Review, in the AI section, algorithms are referred to as blackbox and not easily understood by human-beings [13].

IC is shared decision-making; the informed consent model [ICM] is built on the initial assessment using a bio-psycho-social screening conducted by the primary physician. In most cases, patients must know more about what they agree to when signing off. To ensure the patient's autonomy, the provider must assess that the patient does not have a misguided perception, and even then, it may not be considered a shared effort or even ethical [18].

In a study, *this wasn't a split second,* with youth 14–18-years-of-age, the youth stated that they conducted thorough research on the internet. Some cross referenced their findings with their physician to ensure that what they read was correct information. Other youth stated that if they did not have support and access to GAC that they probably would not be alive today. The IC model of care places the self-determining choice onto the pediatric patient as a shared exchange between the youth, parent, and clinician, permitting self-agency across decision-making. One provider expressed that the signature on the document indicates the individual has the total capacity to understand. Just because a youth is able to conceptualize regret, does not mean they can recognize the risks involved therefore it is critical to evaluate if they are able to realize the consequences of those risks and felt that some youth were easily influenced by peers [19].

Collaborating on IC may require more than exchanging information between provider and patient. Mental health professionals or providers from specialty areas treating the patient often are not involved, included or added to the IC, but are considered best at engaging patients about GAC. Gender identity for some individuals is on a spectrum, and therefore it may not be solidified but malleable over time. A mental health provider would add this as a concern if they determined that the youth may not fully grasp the consequences [20].

Collaboration between medical and social services and other systems has not been shown to benefit patients or their overall health in a study reviewing 36 studies with the authors using Nvivo 12, a qualitative data analysis. In other studies, collaboration may contribute to lowering health inequities, opening avenues for economically disadvantaged patients to access services to mental health care. Partnering improves efficiency, but comes with the challenges of coordinating care and services and gatekeeping within systems not willing to share resources and knowledge [21].

4. Risk management and its' role in identifying risks

Risk management's role in the healthcare industry covers many areas. Risk management's role is to identify risks that lead to poor outcomes and death. Contracts are also reviewed to evaluate potential for risk to the corporation. Forecasting is also part of the assessment. Hospitals that rely on accreditation through Joint Commission are called to a higher standard and benefit when they do not operate as silos [22].

While staff have different roles and responsibilities, in surgical procedures, the nurse, nurse anesthetists, anesthesiologist, scrub nurse, surgeon, are some of the key people who must ensure that the patient is informed every step of the way, is safe, in proper hands, monitored throughout surgery and post surgery, and none of this is possible without teamwork. All steps must have checks and balances. Checklists must be utilized. Overlooking a simple step, such as verifying the patient's name could result in a serious outcome [23].

4.1 Disclosing surgical complications and risks of mortality in the informed consent

A 25-year-old trans man from Georgia passed away from sepsis post-hysterectomy. The reported estimate of percentages of those who develop serious life-threatening complications post hysterectomy in a 2013 study showed a data range between 10.5–9% hinging on the type of surgical approach. The abdominal route carries the highest complication, the vaginal route falls in midrange and laparoscopic hysterectomy has the lowest complications. While over 600,000 hysterectomies are performed annually, death rates are 1% [24]. In the U.S., over half of the hysterectomies are performed via the abdominal route due to a large number of gynecologists not having enough advanced training in laparoscopic procedures while in residency. The abdominal route is the easiest to perform, and improving skill and technique would require performing up to 50 surgical volumes. Still, to date, the average gynecologist may perform no more than 15 cases [25].

A 45-year-old trans male with a history of Factor V Leiden deficiency, Guillain Barre, infective endocarditis, caused by bacteria with a history of drug use, developed postoperative penile artery thrombosis [blood clot], among other complications post phalloplasty. The authors concluded that more research is needed on complications in these surgeries [26].

Dr. Burt Webb, a highly trained gender surgeon recommends that surgeons need at minimum ten years of experience performing phalloplasty surgery [24].

Black TGD population and White TGD population in private insurance between 2011 and 2019 were compared to Black cisgender population and White cisgender population. The findings were not without some setbacks that mainly included individuals who were not out publicly and so did not get counted in as transgender. However, the findings showed inequities in mortality risks among Black TGD people. Black TGD female assigned male at birth were more likely to die at higher rates than Black TGD males and even higher rates as Black cisgender males and females [27].

The most common phalloplasty complication has an incidence of 10–64%. The urethral complication [UC] with a fistula usually presents postoperatively at six months, with the patient complaining of incomplete voiding and difficulty voiding due to a visible fistula [28].

In 2016, Dutch researchers weighed in on a healthy 16-year-old trans female who was part of a study and developed complications 24 hours post surgery. She died from a bacterial infection, called necrotizing fasciitis during the creation of a neovagina using the patient's intestines. This patient had underdeveloped genitals from taking puberty blockers and died days later after large doses of IV antibiotic treatments, repeated wound debridement and went into organ failure. The researchers concluded that the puberty suppression is what caused her demise [29].

A 24-year-old transgender female without any medical comorbidities presented with complaints of fecal matter leaking from her vagina three months post penal flap vaginoplasty. She was followed for two months without any intervention. She was diagnosed with a recto neo-vaginal fistula. The fecal matter was redirected through a Transverse end colostomy until healing occurred and the fistula was later repaired with success [30].

Increasing numbers of complications pertaining to genital surgeries are on the rise. In a study done on Truven MarketScan Database reviewing inpatient and outpatient claims, ICD-9 codes were analyzed for keywords that included breast augmentation, mastectomy, vaginoplasty and phalloplasty. Overall, 1047 insured patients with mastectomy as the most common and phalloplasty as the least common procedure performed. Sixty two complications were reported or 5.8% with wound infection listed as the most common complication and the highest complications came in for phalloplasty surgery [31].

Medical errors in the U.S. are not added to the death certificate. The CDC has listed that some causes of death are due to communication breakdowns between patients, doctors, specialists, and mental health providers, including a lack of adequate volumes in medical care and no follow-up [32].

4.1.1 Disclosing volumes in the informed consent

Patients who suffered injuries have filed lawsuits and wished they had knowledge about the provider's experience and competency. The success of a procedure, some legalists weigh in, hinges on the provider's expertise [33].

Surgeons must be transparent in areas of their expertise during the IC process. Most people obtain this information from others within their community, not via medical vehicles or the surgeon. It is an ethical problem that surgeons omit disclosing how much training they had to perform some of the surgeries [1].

Some researchers argue that the surgical profession needs to provide information about the surgeon's level of expertise and the volume of cases the surgeon has treated [9].

In trauma cases unrelated to GACS, the association between physician volume and patient mortality was made and the authors concluded that higher case volumes were associated with lower mortality [34].

In an oral presentation at the American Urogynecologic Society, Pelvic Floor Disorders Week in October of 2020 and at the Virtual Experience in November of the same year at an oral presentation at WPATHs Virtual Scientific Symposium, the authors of a study determined that neourethral complications in patients receiving asynchronous hysterectomy were possibly due to the inexperience of the surgeon. The authors concluded that two stage steps slightly raised the risk for complications opposed to performing a hysterectomy along with phalloplasty [35].

High rates of urethral stricture disease occur post-metoidioplasty but are much higher with phalloplasty due to the lack of corpora that ordinarily would provide blood flow in cisgender males. Experienced and highly competent surgeons use methods to reduce the odds of urethral constrictions. In contrast, an inexperienced surgeon would cause undue harm and leave the patient with a significant risk of developing strictures and fistulas in these two procedures. Experienced surgeons in GAS have clarified that common repairs occur with strictures at higher recurrence rates and complications as high as 51% than those in cisgender men and stressed that long-term quality data is needed [28].

In a multivariate analysis, penile flap inversion surgical procedures for young trans females with bleeding complications were correlated to the surgeons' clinical and surgical experience. The authors looked at learning curves on the amount of time taken to complete surgery in light of perioperative complications. The authors determined that while this procedure was relatively safe, the younger patient was more challenging due to increase in pelvic muscles and tissue turgor. Operating time was reduced after 22 surgeries for penile flap inversion and even more so after 76 surgeries. The multivariate analysis showed that for vaginal depth, accumulative complications peaked after 32 surgeries and then declined. The authors concluded that surgical experience improved after 30 surgeries. This study was done on one surgeon and the authors expressed that more of these studies are needed on less experienced surgeons for a comparative analysis [36].

According to UCSF Transgender Care, 12% of masculinizing chest surgeries end in complications and are rare for hematoma and infection. The surgical procedure ranges from 2 to 4 hours in duration and hinges on the plastic surgeon's expertise and the patient's physique and composition. Hematomas occur early on and may require reoperation [37].

When hospital surgeons have higher volumes of cases, it speaks to the number of experiences they had performing procedures. A hospital rating is insufficient and will not show the volume of cases the surgeon performed. The connection between volumes and experiences was examined, and the correlation was evident for the risk of death [38].

In an online article by thehealthy.com, Crouch, M., writes about the secrets surgeons withhold from their patients. At Columbia University, Advincula, A., M.D. encourages patients to ask about the surgeon's complication rate but cautions be wary if the surgeon downplays or denies any, because it probably means they have not had enough cases or they are not disclosing the truth. Advincula also emphasizes that some surgeons will not disclose if they know how to perform a type of surgery [39].

In one study on trauma cases, the association between physician volume and patient mortality concluded that higher case volumes were associated with lower mortality [32].

In chapter 22 of Saylor Academy's book on insurance, Medicare, Medicaid, PPOs, HMOs, and individual practice association for Physicians [IPAs] are just some of the insurance plans that have gatekeepers. Gatekeepers who must approve drugs, supplies, durable medical equipment, specialists, and surgeries [40].

4.1.2 Disclosing training in the informed consent

Education for GAS is needed and the estimated time allotted annually is one hour. Slightly over half and under 70% of subjects who participated in a poll stated they were not comfortable with GAS and facial surgery since they had not received much surgical training while 83% recommended increasing the surgical volumes so they could become proficient at GAS [41].

Surgeons providing GAS do not necessarily have the expertise or volumes in areas when performing surgical procedures. Unlike any other type of medical or surgical intervention, physicians and surgeons must have the training and continuous education, but medical or surgical competence is not inherently transparent. Gender affirming surgeries need to be included in medical residency. Masculinizing surgical procedure is an area that needs attention since urethral complications in masculinizing genital surgery range from 25 to 75%. In one case a patient ended up in surgical ICU because he did not disclose his medical history and the treating surgeon and staff who saved his life had to request his records [42, 43].

Genital surgeries require that surgeons have expertise, adequate training in this area, volumes of cases, and collaborative care. Hence, everyone on the team addresses the holistic person's needs, ranging from providing support across many layers inside and outside the family [44].

4.1.3 Research to inform the informed consent

Research paves the way to identify potential problems, life-threatening events, and unforeseen consequences. These guidelines have been included in WPATHs standards of care. We need more input from the TGD individuals with lived experience [45].

Research is needed to inform clear guidelines on supporting detransitioners reversing all or parts of this process. Dr. Kinnon MacKinnon points out that there are insufficient numbers to know how many individuals have detransitioned and recommends setting goals to reduce stress for detransitioners and that longitudinal studies are needed. Some WPATH leaders are concerned and have expressed the need to learn from the detransitioners to better serve the transgender population [46].

In Germany, an analysis was conducted on the quality of ICs unrelated to GACS. Ten forms of medical treatments' content were analyzed in 14 areas and determined to be insufficient in evaluating important areas, risks, and benefits and for the opting out of procedures and treatment, among others but overall found sufficient evidence that ICs did not support an informed decision. Thirty-seven informed consents were reviewed from publishers and practices throughout Germany. Regulations in Germany call for a model professional code for physicians to engage in pre-discussions before treatment [47].

In the Open Letter to WPATH community members strongly recommended that WPATH consider an advisory board of patients with lived experience to inform surgical guidelines [3].

Guidelines are developed through a consensus process led by TGD experts that prevent harm, improve the patient's well-being, and address any medical and mental health concerns to provide quality care to the individual [6].

Guidelines are developed without input from those with lived experience. Funding is needed for research and quality measures and outcomes to advance best practices [3].

Research is lacking, and there are currently no clear guidelines on supporting detransitioners reversing all or parts of this process. There are insufficient numbers to know how many have detransitioned or recommend setting goals to reduce stress for detransitioners. In an online survey on 237 detransitioners most of their gender dysphoria related to other comorbidities that ranged from PTSD to ADHD [48].

4.2 Research to inform training

In the Open Letter by community members having undergone GAS sent to WPATH call for research on learning curves and only granting surgeons accreditation after completely satisfying supervised number of hours and procedures. The members reported concerns with WPATH surgeons with insufficient training capitalizing on building volume by offering free or low-cost surgeries to under-resourced patients. Patients reported feeling abandoned in aftercare among misstatements by board-certified plastic surgeons who dismissed knowledge about nerve coaptation [3].

Medical residents need a full-fledged educational curriculum in their surgical program for gender-affirming surgical procedures that range from facial feminization to feminizing and masculinizing genitalia surgical procedures. Residency training is needed because many residents do not feel adequately prepared [49].

5. Accreditation in gender-affirming care

Joint Commission has raised concerns with ICs and reports that IC is compromised and protects the providers, and is not sufficiently informing the patient without discussion. Joint Commission cites a study from 2016 that reported four essential elements were left out in 26.4 percent of the ICs. The fourth element included the alternatives to medical or surgical treatment. Between 2010 and 2021, 1.3% of reported cases received wrong-site surgical procedures and six cases were related to operative and post operative complications according to Joint Commission's Sentinel Event Database. A sentinel event results in semi or permanent harm to a patient, such as near death or death. A Sentinel Event in Joint Commission's report calls for immediate investigation because the event is a serious adverse outcome. Medical errors are the second leading cause of death, creating a serious public health problem [50, 51].

Joint Commission in 2020 published an article on patient's reporting adverse events and harm caused by their health care provider. Joint Commission deemed these as significant and identified surgical/medication events, hospital-acquired infection, diagnostic error as some of the types of harm. One of the contributing factors listed the patient had not received sufficient information to make an informed decision [52].

Safety and regret are synonymous when the outcomes result in depression, suicidal ideation, and attempted suicide. Healthcare professionals also suffer, and no data exist on physicians taking their lives because of botched procedures, possibly because professionals fear retaliation and reluctance to report errors or patient regret [53].

In a seminal study from 1990, Joint Commission was created in 1951 for the purpose to accredit hospitals to meet safety standards, recognize the pitfalls of IC serving as a piece of paper for a patient to sign without any discussion and that, too many times, patients do not fully understand what risks and benefits entail. In the PROs and CONs section of the study, the downside of accrediting a process is the limited availability of surveyors from professional agencies. The other downside is when there is noncompliance, the accreditation is not a guarantee until it has been proven that conditions were met. Additional impediments were listed in the conclusions of quality assurance through certification and accreditation that set federal standards of care. Accreditation agencies are important in healthcare. They ensure that agencies and hospitals meet the highest quality of care and safety standards so patients can make informed decisions [54].

5.1 Detransitioners and AI

In a mixed method analysis codes were classified as external factors from internal factors on detransitioners. Vast majority reported it was due to external factors, pressures to fit in society, having to take care of a loved one, not feeling safe at work with some due to internal factors among others. The authors expressed that these could have run interference with the aide of a mental health provider. Trans females were more likely to detransition [55].

Detransitioners are speaking out about their experiences. In an article in Reuters titled *Why detransitioners are crucial to the science of gender care*, some transgender rights activists are at odds with detransitioners and express that detransitioners are underhanded and creating problems for the trans community. A lead at the Amsterdam University Centre for Expertise on Gender Dysphoria encourages everyone to listen to these narratives as these afford a time of reflection on what we have learned so far and what we need to know to improve care. Detransitioners reported mental health co-morbidities as teenagers [47].

One study concluded that barriers exist in pediatricians who may lack the expertise to care for TGD youth. Fifty caregivers and 15 youths were dissatisfied with services due to inconsistent care and lack of cultural competency. They expressed concerns about gatekeeping and delays in accessing medical treatment for blockers and hormones [56].

Some transgender and gender diverse [TGD] individuals reported regret in several areas ranging from misdiagnosis and hormonal transition to post-surgical regret. Guardian released an article by Rachel Cooke on British Broadcasting Corporation [BBC] journalist Hannah Barnes's book titled *Time to Think.* England's Tavistock's gender identity clinic changed the informed consent [IC] process from its original intent to provide support for gender development. In the fifth column of the article, the clinic's revenue grew as more and more children and adolescents were seen and treated by providers with little to no expertise in prescribing puberty blockers and gender-affirming hormonal treatment [GAHT]. In addition, complaints were filed for a lack of follow-up care, and lack of data entering and tracking on cases seen and treated through the clinic [57].

Pressure on providers to meet the demands in responding to the growth in GAC has led to some providers treating GAC as the standard of care with some lacking the expertise to evaluate youth [6].

The concerns over time with delays in treatment for GAS led to a revision in WPATHs SOC8. WPATH offers a gold standard for guidelines. In the frequently asked question section of SOC8, WPATHs revised guidelines now recommend only one letter of recommendation [LOR] versus two [4].

A retrospective audit was conducted on all new patients seeking GAHT who reported great satisfaction with their general practitioner and 80 percent of 43 participants in a survey chose a mental health provider for support while nine others did not. The conclusion in this audit deemed quicker access to care and lower wait times as part of the reason in addition to participants choosing a mental health provider [58].

A physician who takes the time to evaluate, investigate, and rule out the patient's diagnosis can reduce the likelihood of liability. Unfortunately, a study showed that doctors interrupt the patient within 11 seconds [59].

The Accreditation Council for Graduate Medical Education [ACGME] committee opinion reviewed communication among OBGYNE doctors. ACGME identified physicians as needing training in communication as it has been shown to improve patient outcomes. Several models to improve communication served as examples [60].

In a systemic review on post-surgical regret, in a section titled *Reasons for Regret*, 10 out of 14 patients opted to detransition surgically. These individuals expressed social regret or inwardly feeling a deep sense of regret or no longer identified as male or female but somewhere in between [61].

Given the uncertainty and lack of reported outcomes, medicalizing a condition as part of development is risky. A study on a population of 100 detransitioners revealed that those who detransitioned did so because of stigmatization, unsatisfactory surgical results, realizing that they were struggling with homophobia, adverse reaction to GAHT, and reidentifying with their natal sex [62].

Claims of puberty-blocking agents have been made reversible without unsupported evidence, and the natural experience for an adolescent to experience puberty is disrupted [63]. A qualitative study using constructivist grounded theory reported that 28 Canadian adults who transitioned did so without regret but avoided any follow-up with their clinician to prevent stigma because the clinician lacked clinical knowledge in this area [64, 65].

Some scholars determine that a diagnosis for gender incongruence is of poor quality with mistaken assumptions about the patient in providing gender-affirming treatment and surgery [GATS]. Patients, caregivers, and parents receive incomplete or inaccurate information and even disinformation that if a child or teen does not receive gender-affirming care [GAC], this will lead to suicide. Mistaken assumptions, incomplete or erroneous information, and disinformation are all fueled by the rise in individuals seeking GACS and GAT. Protocols are lacking for individuals who identify as non-binary or who seek micro-dosing to qualify for hormonal treatment. The IC lacks certainty because the focus is more on gender dysphoria as opposed to what may lie behind this diagnosis, as in some cases of regret, patients realized that it had more to do with their mental illness than it did with gender dysphoria [6].

One study concluded that barriers exist in pediatricians who may lack the expertise to care for TGD youth. Fifty caregivers and 15 youths were dissatisfied with services due to inconsistent care and lack of cultural competency. They expressed concerns about gatekeeping and delays in accessing medical treatment for blockers and hormones [57].

5.2 The cost of transgender care

Volumes in GAS are growing, but adding a multidisciplinary team would build an integrated process strictly devoted to a multitude of interventions ranging from mental health care, to providers involved in the patient's care prior to transitioning to surgical services and follow-up care for any concerns, complications, or revisions [66].

High costs may hamper GAS and is on demand. Its projected value for 2032 is USD 1.9 billion. The GAS market size in Europe is estimated to rise above 482 million. The market index shows an 11% growth from 2020 to 2021 for GAS, with revenue reported as $1.9 billion. Mount Sinai Center for Transgender Medicine and Surgery performed 639 female gender affirming surgeries [fGAS], 222 volumes above transgender male affirming surgeries [mGAS] [66, 67].

Prediction models by design help patients and physicians make patient-tailored decisions, as evidenced in a Thoracic Surgery Evaluation and Treatment model. Prediction models focus on variables that could predict negative and positive outcomes. These outcomes help facilitate a shared decision-making between patient and the provider. Some of the prediction models can calculate a patient's surgical risks [68].

When malpractice suits are filed because the surgeon failed to disclose their inexperience and the risks, the informed consent in a number of these cases was not considered adequate and was deemed to have failed the patient [69].

6. Conclusion

As with any other specialty, GAS warrants cycling through a vigorous accreditation process. Acknowledgment that higher volumes are linked to better outcomes indicates that surgeons must perform many surgeries before they are considered eligible to perform a procedure. Surgical residencies need to offer GAS and surgeons seeking experience should be required to meet a standard established by experts. Surgeons must comply and meet the educational requirements and experience in number of volumes. Patients need follow-up care and revisions to address complications post-surgery. The Open Letter to WPATH clearly signals a disturbing pattern with patient abandonment post surgery. As the Open Letter addresses concerns with lack of oversight and lack of competency, WPATH could collaborate with TGD individuals whose lived experience would best inform needed surgical policies and procedures for pre and post care, training, and oversight. The IC is limiting and needs to include the surgeons expertise and training.

WPATH offers certification to members in good standing. Insisting on certification and vigorous training before surgeons can operate necessitates oversight. Seeking accreditation may benefit WPATH. Programs that seek Joint Commission accreditation benefit as this elevates the organization's credentials, however the downside is the limited availability of surveyors from professional agencies that oversee accreditation.

Adverse events are not tracked in gender-affirming care as there are no guidelines for what constitutes an adverse event and when to report one. To say that complications are rare is a bit premature given we do not have enough data. Some of the data is skewed given the different descriptive words used for conditions.

The insurance industry has information that is valuable and could inform patterns in areas of competency with surgeons, number of surgical revisions typical and atypical among surgeons and ratings of outcomes among surgeons. Insurance companies are gatekeepers and the idea that the IC needs to avoid gatekeeping is erroneous. The IC over time has deteriorated to nothing but a piece of paper warranting the patient's signature but very little effort is placed on protecting the patient's best interest.

Some surgeons are not WPATH members and do not require the person to have a letter of recommendation [LOR] for GAS that is opposite of what WPATH SOC8 recommends. WPATH could consider collaborating with a legislative body to require that all surgeons must adhere to WPATH standards. Regulatory bodies could work with the insurance industry and require LORs before surgeons can perform GAS.

Preexisting conditions could prove to be fatal if not addressed prior to implementing GAC. IC could list patients' potential risk factors using electronic data records. While a number of gender surgery centres with high volume cases review patient's history, this may not be in the case of the surgeon owning their own surgical centres, with little to no experience, scheduled to perform phalloplasty or vaginoplasty. TGD care is a specialty.

Knowing a doctor's experience helps patients determine if they can risk opting for treatment or surgery, forego both and opt for alternatives instead. Doctors need to supply their patients with alternative information responsibly.

The consensus is lacking for AI development in identifying individuals with a propensity for detransitioning that may have been intercepted early on if several factors were in place. Utilizing codes for detransitioners from surveys and translating these into AI could filter through predictive indicators reported by detransitioners to determine whether the individual needs guidance and support for typologies associated with a propensity for depression or complications due to medical preconditions. The downside of AI is the assumption that everyone is alike when two people present with a clean bill of health but the AI focused only on one type of profile. One person undergoing masculinizing genital surgery may end up with regret for a number of reasons that include poor recovery and complications, and the other will have a successful uneventful transition, but the predictability narrows the more experienced the surgeon and with collaborative efforts of others.

Augmenting the IC with a risk prediction model may be beneficial in informing the patient about the risks and benefits based on their preexisting conditions and comorbidities from their electronic [ED] record.

Given we do not have enough data to determine how many other individuals will report they detransitioned because of surgical regret or medical regret, it would be beneficial to require monitoring and keeping track of this data.

Utilizing codes for detransitioners from surveys and translating these into AI could filter through predictive indicators as reported by detransitioners. AI could determine whether the individual needs guidance and support for typologies associated with a propensity for depression or complications due to medical preconditions. AI may be beneficial in linking typologies specific to the patient or their familial history and AI could potentially review risk factors based on the patient's history before deciding on GAC or GAS. The IC is then built upon this model of care that includes comorbid conditions affected by GAHT and GACS. For example, if a patient has a history of a blood clotting disorder and is planning on undergoing phalloplasty or vaginoplasty, coordinating care with hematology or the treating provider, may best serve this patient. Having discussions about GAHT so that the individual has relative information and can opt to seek alternatives if so desired as opposed to the IC only fulfilling the four elements.

Reports of low mortality risks in GAS are questionable given that we need to collect data from systems serving uninsured patients and combine these reports with the insurance industry. Despite reports of low mortality risks in GAS, risk managements' role is vital, such as in the case of patients left abandoned, in need of post surgical care or revision surgery.

When prediction models to gauge patient's surgical risks are not used, patient's such as the gentleman with a history of Guillan Barre and Factor V Leiden may have had a different outcome had one been used to predict his surgical risk. Not having this information readily available, it is difficult to determine if a prediction model was used or if the patient even disclosed his history. If the patient did not disclose his history, but his records were accessed or other clinicians were part of his IC, perhaps they may have added his history and consulted with a hematologist. The reality exists that some patients are poor historians or do not share their medical history.

In the case of patients left with poor outcomes, complications that have posed difficulty for the person to navigate through life, such as the case with a patient who ends up abandoned by the system and cannot afford or is denied a revision, a coordinated team would guide and connect the patient to services. In the case of a detransitioner expressing surgical regret, the doctor's role is to offer alternatives. The role of the mental health provider is to support the person's transition from the beginning through the middle all the way up to the end of the person's transition. But even beyond transition as life events do occur.

Training, education, coordinated care, mental health care, regulation, accreditation, and expanding the IC are just some of the recommendations that could improve GACS in hopes to reduce narratives of regret.

Acronyms

ACGME	Accreditation Council for Graduate Medical Education
AI	artificial intelligence
AMA	American Medical Association

CABP	coronary artery bypass procedure
DNV	Det Norske Veritas
ED	electronic record
FCA	False Claims Act
fGAS	female genital affirming surgery
GACS	gender-affirming care/surgery
GAHT	gender-affirming hormone treatment
GAS	gender-affirming surgery
HRT	hormone replacement therapy
IC	informed consent
IPA	Individual Practice Association
mGAS	male genital-affirming surgery
NCQA	National Committee for Quality Assurance
TGD	transgender-gender diverse
SOC8	standards of care—version 8
UC	urethral complication
WPATH	World Professional Association for Transgender Health

Author details

An Goldbauer
International Institute of Clinical Sexology, Miami Shores, Florida, United States of America

*Address all correspondence to: dr.angoldbauer@gmail.com

IntechOpen

© 2024 The Author(s). Licensee IntechOpen. This chapter is distributed under the terms of the Creative Commons Attribution License (http://creativecommons.org/licenses/by/3.0), which permits unrestricted use, distribution, and reproduction in any medium, provided the original work is properly cited.

References

[1] Boskey ER, Kant JD. Unreasonable expectations: A call for training and educational transparency in gender-affirming surgery. Plastic and Reconstructive Surgery—Global Open. 2023;**11**(1):e4734. Available from: https://journals.lww.com/prsgo/Fulltext/2023/01000/Unreasonable_Expectations__A_Call_for_Training_and.18.aspx

[2] Usnews.com. 2023. Available from: https://health.usnews.com/health-news/blogs/second-opinion/articles/2016-11-18/why-surgical-volumes-should-be-public

[3] WPATHopenletter.wp.com 2018. WPATH open letter. blog at wordpress.com. Available from: https://wpathopenletter.wordpress.com/ [Accessed: May 2, 2023]

[4] World professional association for transgender health standards of care for transgender and gender diverse people, version 8 frequently asked questions (FAQs) what are the world professional association for transgender health's standards of care for transgender and gender diverse people?. Wpath.org. 2023. Available from: https://www.wpath.org/media/cms/Documents/SOC%20v8/SOC-8%20FAQs%20-%20WEBSITE2.pdf

[5] Ziegler E, Valaitis R, Risdon C, Carter N, Yost J. Models of care and team activities in the delivery of transgender primary care: An Ontario case study. Transgender Health. 2020;**5**(2):122-112. Available from: https://www.ncbi.nlm.nih.gov/pmc/articles/PMC7347017/

[6] Levine SB, Abbruzzese E, Mason JW. Reconsidering informed consent for trans identified children, adolescents, and young adults. Journal of Sex & Marital Therapy. 2022;**17**:706-772. Available from: https://www.tandfonline.com/doi/full/10.1080/0092623X.2022.2046221?scroll=top&needAccess=true&role=tab&aria-labelledby=full-article

[7] Informed consent. Ama-assn.org. 2023. Available from: https://code-medical-ethics.ama-assn.org/ethics-opinions/informed-consent

[8] Cocanour C. Informed consent: It's more than a signature on a piece of paper. The American Journal of Surgery. 2018;**214**:993-997. DOI: 10.1016/j.amjsurg.2017.09.015

[9] Burger I, Schill K, Goodman S. Disclosure of individual surgeon's performance rates during informed consent: Ethical and epistemological considerations. Annals of Surgery. 2007;**245**(4):507-551. DOI: 10.1097/01.sla.0000242713.82125.d1

[10] Painter K. Do you check online doctor ratings? 1 in 4 consumers do. USA Today. 2014. Available from: https://www.usatoday.com/story/news/nation/2014/02/18/online-doctor-ratings/5582257/

[11] FSMB. Fsmb.org. Available from: https://www.fsmb.org/fcvs/

[12] André P, Filip A, Moldovan R. Segment disclosure quantity and quality under IFRS 8: Determinants and the effect on financial analysts' earnings forecast errors. The International Journal of Accounting. 2016;**51**(4):443-461

[13] Cohen G, Atwood JA, Williams L. Informed Consent and Medical Artificial Intelligence; What to Tell the Patient? by Georgetown Law Review.

Washington, DC, USA: The Georgetown Law Journal; 2023. pp. 1425-1146. Available from: https://www.law.georgetown.edu/georgetownlaw-journal/wp-content/uploads/sites/26/2020/06/Cohen_Informed-Consent-and-Medical-Artificial-Intelligence-What-to-Tell-the-Patient.pdf

[14] Buck DI. Overtreatment and informed consent: A fraud-based solution to unwanted and unnecessary care. Florida State University Law Review 2017;**43**(3):901-995. Available from: https://www.fsulawreview.com/article/overtreatment-and-informed-consent-a-fraud-based-solution-to-unwanted-and-unnecessary-care/#p929 [Accessed: 2023, May 15]

[15] Pronovost P. Why surgical volumes should be public. Voices for Safer Care | Insights from the Armstrong Institute. Voices for Safer Care; 2016. Available from: https://armstronginstitute.blogs.hopkinsmedicine.org/2016/12/06/why-surgical-volumes-should-be-public/

[16] Surgical volumes. Hopkinsmedicine.org. 2023. Available from: https://www.hopkinsmedicine.org/patient_safety/surgical_volumes.html

[17] Grote T, Berens P. On the ethics of algorithmic decision-making in healthcare. Journal of Medical Ethics. 2020;**46**(3):205-211. Available from: https://jme.bmj.com/content/46/3/205

[18] Gerritse K, Hartman LA, Bremmer MA, Kreukels BPC, Molewijk BC. Decision-making approaches in transgender healthcare: Conceptual analysis and ethical implications. Medicine, Health Care, and Philosophy. 2021;**24**(4):687-699. DOI: 10.1007/s11019-021-10023-6

[19] Clark BA, Virani A. This wasn't a split-second decision: An empirical ethical analysis of transgender youth capacity, rights, and authority to consent to hormone therapy. Journal of Bioethical Inquiry. 2021;**18**(1):151-164. DOI: 10.1007/s11673-020-10086-9

[20] Chiang T, Bachmann GA. The informed consent model is adequate for gender-affirming treatment: Issues related with mental health assessment in the United States. The Journal of Sexual Medicine. 2023;**20**(5):584-587. Available from: https://academic.oup.com/jsm/article/20/5/584/7145730

[21] Alderwick H, Hutchings A, Briggs A, Mays N. The impacts of collaboration between local health care and non-health care organizations and factors shaping how they work: A systematic review of reviews. BMC Public Health. 2021;**21**(1):2-6. DOI: 10.1186/s12889-021-10630-1

[22] Reviews C. Risk Management for Enterprises and Individuals: Business, Management. La Vergne, TN: Cram101; 2016. Available from: https://saylordotorg.github.io/text_risk-management-for-enterprises-and-individuals/index.html

[23] McGowan J, Wojahn A, Nicolini JR. Risk Management Event Evaluation and Responsibilities. Treasure Island, Florida: StatPearls Publishing; 2023

[24] Trans man's death sparks questions about the safety of hysterectomy. Hysto.net. Available from: https://www.hysto.net/hysterectomy-safety.htm

[25] Hysterectomy options. Brighamandwomens.org. Available from: https://www.brighamandwomens.org/obgyn/minimally-invasive-gynecologic-surgery/hysterectomy-options

[26] Gilbert Z, Markovic JP, Stultz D. Phalloplasty complicated by penile artery

thrombosis, recurrent extended-spectrum beta-lactamase (ESBL) urinary tract infection (UTI), colovesical fistula, and enterococcus faecalis endocarditis. Cureus. 2021;**13**(11):e19716. Available from: https://www.cureus.com/articles/63922-phalloplasty-complicated-by-penile-artery-thrombosis-recurrent-extended-spectrum-beta-lactamase-esbl-urinary-tract-infection-uti-colovesical-fistula-and-enterococcus-faecalis-endocarditis#!/

[27] Hughes LD, King WM, Gamarel KE, Geronimus AT, Panagiotou OA, Hughto JMW. US Black-White differences in mortality risk among transgender and cisgender people in private insurance, 2011-2019. American Journal of Public Health. 2022;**112**(10):1507-1514. DOI: 10.2105/AJPH.2022.306963

[28] Jun MS, Santucci RA. Urethral stricture after phalloplasty. Translational Andrology and Urology. 2019;**8**(3):266-272. DOI: 10.21037/tau.2019.05.08

[29] Soniya Y. Transgender teenager dies after vaginoplasty surgery goes awfully wrong. Sportskeeda. 2023. Available from: https://www.sportskeeda.com/health-and-fitness/transgender-teenager-dies-vaginoplasty-surgery-goes-awfully-wrong

[30] Omarov N, Tatar S. The repairing of the recto-neovaginal fistula in a male-to-female transgender through perineal graciloplasty. Cureus. 2021;**13**(6):e15784. DOI: 10.7759/cureus.15784

[31] Lane M, Ives GC, Sluiter EC, Waljee JF, Yao T-H, Hu HM, et al. Trends in gender-affirming surgery in insured patients in the United States. Plastic and Reconstructive Surgery. Global Open. 2018;**6**(4):e1738. DOI: 10.1097/GOX.0000000000001738

[32] Makary MA, Daniel M. Medical error—The third leading cause of death in the US. BMJ. 2016;**353**:i2139. Available from: https://www.bmj.com/content/353/bmj.i2139.full

[33] Cohen G, Elhauge E, Gilman D, Keefe T, Koch VG, Mehlman M, et al. Modernizing informed consent: Expanding the boundaries of materiality. Illinoislawreview.org. 838 p. Available from: https://www.illinoislawreview.org/wp-content/uploads/2016/07/Sawicki.pdf

[34] Saviluoto A, Pappinen J, Kirves H, Raatiniemi L, Nurmi J. Association between physician's case volume in prehospital advanced trauma care and 30-day mortality: A registry-based analysis of 4,032 patients. The Journal of Trauma and Acute Care Surgery. 2023;**94**(3):425-432. Available from: https://journals.lww.com/jtrauma/Fulltext/2023/03000/Association_between_physician_s_case_volume_in.10.aspx

[35] Ha B, Morrill MY, Salim AM, Stram D, Weiss E. Differences in surgical complications for stage 1 phalloplasty with concurrent versus asynchronous hysterectomy in transmasculine patients. The Permanente Journal. 2022;**26**(4):49-55. DOI: 10.7812/TPP/22.054

[36] Maurer V, Howaldt M, Feldmann I, Ludwig T, Vetterlein MW, Gild P, et al. Penile flap inversion vaginoplasty in transgender women: Contemporary morbidity and learning-curve analysis from a high-volume reconstructive center. Frontiers in Surgery. 2022;**9**(2022):836335. Available from: https://www.frontiersin.org/articles/10.3389/fsurg.2022.836335/full

[37] Postoperative care and common issues after masculinizing chest surgery. Ucsf.edu. Available from: https://transcare.ucsf.edu/guidelines/chest-surgery-masculinizing

[38] Gregory J. Making hospital—Surgical volume data public. Healthexec.com. 2016. Available from: https://healthexec.com/topics/healthcare-management/healthcare-quality/making-hospital-level-surgical-volume-data-public

[39] Crouch M. The Healthy Magazine. 2021. Available from: https://www.thehealthy.com/healthcare/doctors/50-secrets-your-surgeon-wont-tell-you/

[40] Insurance Services Office, Inc. Risk Management for Enterprises and Individuals. Available from: https://saylordotorg.github.io/text_risk-management-for-enterprises-and-individuals/index.html

[41] Morris MM, Llado-Farrulla MM, Christopher AN, Patel V, Broach RB, Percec I. Gender-affirming surgery in plastic surgery. 2021;**9**(10s):113-114. Available from: https://journals.lww.com/prsgo/Fulltext/2021/10001/Gender_affirming_Surgery_in_Plastic_Surgery.154.aspx

[42] Mani VR, Valdivieso SC, Hanandeh A, Kalabin A, Ramcharan A, Donaldson B. Transgender surgery-knowledge gap among physicians impacting patient care. Current Urology. 2021;**15**(1):68-70

[43] Kelly-Schuette K, Little A, Davis AT, Mensah FK, Wright GP. Transgender surgery: Perspectives across levels of training in medical and surgical specialties. Transgender Health. 2021;**6**(4):217-223. Available from: https://www.ncbi.nlm.nih.gov/pmc/articles/PMC8363995

[44] Aquino NJ, Boskey ER, Staffa SJ, et al. A single center case series of gender-affirming surgeries and the evolution of a specialty anesthesia team. Journal of Clinical Medicine. 2022;**11**(7):1943. DOI: 10.3390/jcm11071943

[45] Veale J, Deutsch M, Radix A, Devor A, Motmans J, St. Amand, Colton. Setting a research agenda in trans health: An expert assessment of priorities and issues by trans and nonbinary researchers. International Journal of Transgender Health. 2022;**23**(4):392-408. DOI: 10.1080/26895269.2022.2044425

[46] Robin respaut CTAMC. Why detransitioners are crucial to the science of gender care. Reuters. 2022. Available from: https://www.reuters.com/investigates/special-report/usa-transyouth-outcomes/

[47] Lühnen J, Mühlhauser I, Steckelberg A. The Quality of Informed Consent Forms-a Systematic Review and Critical Analysis. Dtsch Arztebl Int. 2018 Jun 1;**115**(22):377-383. DOI: 10.3238/arztebl.2018.0377. PMID: 29932049; PMCID: PMC6039714

[48] Irwig MS. Detransition among transgender and gender-diverse people-an increasing and increasingly complex phenomenon. The Journal of Clinical Endocrinology and Metabolism. 2022;**107**(10):e4261-e4262. Available from: https://academic.oup.com/jcem/article/107/10/e4261/6604653

[49] Mousavian M, Ranganathan K, Kumar A. State of educational modalities employed in gender-affirming surgery amongst surgical residencies. Global Surgical Education. 2022;**1**(1):1-10. DOI: 10.1007/s44186-022-00065-6

[50] Quick Safety 21: Informed consent: More than getting a signature (Updated: April 2022). Jointcommission.org. Available from: https://www.jointcommission.org/resources/news-and-multimedia/newsletters/newsletters/quick-safety/quick-safety--issue-21-informed--consent-more-than-getting-a-signature/informed-consent-more-than-getting-a-signature/

[51] Sentinel Event Policy and procedures. Jointcommission.org. Available from: https://www.jointcommission.org/resources/sentinel-event/sentinel-event-policy-and-procedures/

[52] Jointcommissionjournal.com. Available from: https://www.jointcommissionjournal.com/article/S1553-7250(20)30036-2/pdf

[53] Rodziewicz TL, Houseman B, Hipskind JE. Medical Error Reduction and Prevention. StatPearls [Internet] Treasure Island, Florida: StatPearls Publishing; 2023. Available from: https://www.ncbi.nlm.nih.gov/books/NBK499956/

[54] Lohr KN. Medicare Conditions of Participation and Accreditation for Hospitals. Washington, DC: National Academies Press; 1990

[55] Turban JL, Loo SS, Almazan AN, Keuroghlian AS. Factors leading to "detransition" among transgender and gender diverse people in the United States: A mixed-methods analysis. LGBT Health. 2021;**8**(4):273-280. DOI: 10.1089/lgbt.2020.0437

[56] Gridley SJ, Crouch JM, Evans Y, Eng W, Antoon E, Lyapustina M, et al. Youth and caregiver perspectives on barriers to gender-affirming health care for transgender youth. The Journal of Adolescent Health. 2016;**59**(3):254-261. DOI: 10.1016/j.jadohealth.2016.03.017

[57] Cooke R. Time to think by Hannah Barnes review – What went wrong at Gids? The Guardian. 2023. Available from: https://www.theguardian.com/books/2023/feb/19/time-to-think-by-hannah-barnes-review-what-went-wrong-at-gids

[58] Spanos C, Grace JA, Leemaqz SY, Brownhill A, Cundill P, Locke P, et al. The informed consent model of care for accessing gender-affirming hormone therapy is associated with high patient satisfaction. The Journal of Sexual Medicine. 2021;**18**(1):201-208. DOI: 10.1016/j.jsxm.2020.10.020

[59] Phillips KA, Ospina NS, Montori VM. Physicians interrupting patients. Journal of General Internal Medicine. 2019;**34**(10):1965. DOI: 10.1007/s11606-019-05247-5

[60] Available from: https://www.acog.org/-/media/project/acog/acogorg/clinical/files/committee-opinion/articles/2014/02/effective-patient-physician-communication.pdf

[61] Bustos VP, Bustos SS, Mascaro A, Del Corral G, Forte AJ, Ciudad P, et al. Regret after gender-affirmation surgery: A systematic review and meta-analysis of prevalence. Plastic and Reconstructive Surgery. Global Open. 2021;**9**(3):e3477. DOI: 10.1097/GOX.0000000000003477

[62] Littman L. Individuals treated for gender dysphoria with medical and/or surgical transition who subsequently detransitioned: A survey of 100 detransitioners. Archives of Sexual Behavior. 2021;**50**(8):3353-3369. DOI: 10.1007/s10508-021-02163-w

[63] Hayes K. Ethical implications of treatment for gender dysphoria in youth. Online Journal of Health Ethics. 2018;**14**(2):6, 8-10. Available from: https://aquila.usm.edu/cgi/viewcontent.cgi?article=1214&context=ojhe

[64] MacKinnon KR, Kia H, Salway T, Ashley F, Lacombe-Duncan A, Abramovich A, et al. Health care experiences of patients discontinuing or reversing prior gender-affirming treatments. JAMA Network Open. 2022;**5**(7):e2224717. DOI: 10.1001/jamanetworkopen.2022.24717

[65] Manrique OJ, Bustos SS, Bustos VP, Mascaro AA, Ciudad P, Forte AJ, et al. Building a multidisciplinary academic surgical gender-affirmation program: Lessons learned. Plastic and Reconstructive Surgery. Global Open. 2021;**9**(3):e3478. DOI: 10.1097/GOX.0000000000003478

[66] U.S. Sex Reassignment Surgery Market Size, Share & Trends Analysis Report by Gender Transition (Male To Female, Female To Male), And Segment Forecasts. 2022-2030. Available from: https://www.grandviewresearch.com/industry-analysis/us-sex-reassignment-surgery-market

[67] Sex Reassignment Surgery Market. 2023. Available from: https://www.gminsights.com/industry-analysis/sex-reassignment-surgery-market

[68] Shipe ME, Deppen SA, Farjah F, Grogan EL. Developing prediction models for clinical use using logistic regression: An overview. Journal of Thoracic Disease. 2019;**11**(Suppl. 4): S574-S584. Available from: https://jtd.amegroups.com/article/view/26585/html

[69] Iheukwumere EO. Doctor, are ye You Experienced? The Relevance of Disclosure of Physician Experience to a vo a Valid Informed Consent. Law.edu. Available from: https://scholarship.law.edu/cgi/viewcontent.cgi?article=1215&context=jchlp

Chapter 4

Fentanyl and Its Derivatives, Pharmacology, Use and Abuse, and Detection Possibilities

Romana Jelínková

Abstract

The chapter presents one of the most discussed synthetic anesthetics—fentanyl. The possibilities of its use, the effect on the health of users, pharmacological and chemical findings, the issue of human and veterinary use of these substances, and the comparison of the effects of its derivatives are described. It discusses the issue of the abuse of these psychoactive substances and their seizures by members of the rescue system and the necessity of legislative control. Some methods of detecting fentanyl-type substances are listed, both by simple orientation methods and by more sophisticated techniques of infrared spectroscopy and liquid and gas chromatography. Finally, fentanyl is discussed as an incapacitating agent in the protection of the population.

Keywords: fentanyl, pharmacology, chemical properties, instrumental detection, Kolokol-1

1. Introduction

The existence of pain-relieving substances has been known since ancient times. The first opioid analgesics were probably natural alkaloids found in the poppy. Morphine was isolated from poppy opium, which was successfully used as a powerful analgesic and sedative. At the end of the nineteenth century, pharmaceutical companies began to focus on the synthesis of new effective drugs.

The story of the most popular opioid analgesic, fentanyl, dates back to 1959, when Dr. Paul Janssen, pharmacologist, physician, and founder of Janssen Pharmaceutica, sought an adequate substitute for the opioid pethidine (also called meperidine, trade name Demerol). The pethidine used at the time showed weak analgesic effects compared to morphine. Due to its simple molecule structure Dr. Janssen assumed that by changing the pethidine structure and achieving better solubility in fats, the newly synthesized substance would have a stronger effect on the organism. Selected opioids have previously been used in anesthetic care for premedication, as intraoperative adjuncts to general anesthesia, and for postoperative pain management.

From a number of newly synthesized molecular entities that showed significant analgesic activity, a substance called fentanyl appeared to be the most advantageous, the effects of which being about 80–100 times stronger than those of morphine.

IntechOpen

Subsequently, numerous experiments were carried out on animals, first in combination with other inhaled drugs and later as a pure narcotic anesthetic.

Based on the positive results, studies were started in Europe, and fentanyl was approved for regular use in medical practice in the mid-1860s. It was usually used to put people to sleep in combination with some intravenously administered hypnotics, such as droperidol. This technique of "neurolept anesthesia" soon gained considerable popularity. The states of analgesia, apathy, and deep sedation—the neurolept-analgesia, when the patient can be awakened and when the patient can speak, and neuroleptanesthesia, in which the patient is unconscious, are procedures that allow short and medium-term surgical and diagnostic procedures in patients with cardiovascular diseases with minimal load on the heart and circulatory system. Later, the combination of fentanyl with droperidol was replaced by a combination of fentanyl or alfentanil with a benzodiazepine due to differences in the pharmacokinetics of these substances [1].

The effect of fentanyl is qualitatively similar to morphine. Cortical depression has been shown to be minimal, and respiratory changes may outlast its analgesic effect. However, no significant cardiovascular effects were observed at usual therapeutic doses [2]. The advantage is a lower emetic effect compared to morphine [3].

After its introduction as an intravenous analgesic, it was used in a number of Western European countries in combination with other sedatives or hypnotics in an attempt to create a unique general intravenous anesthesia. Due to its high efficiency, it was possible to use only a minimal amount of the substance [4]. Throughout Europe, "neurolept anesthesia" was subsequently studied for more than a quarter of a century as an alternative to the strong inhalation anesthetics of the time. At the turn of the 1960s and 1970s, the so-called "stress-free anesthesia" came to the fore in Belgium thanks to the anesthesiologist Gorge de Castro and the Janssen team. Stress-free anesthesia refers to the use of a drug or combination of drugs that can provide deep anesthesia with minimal or no change in cardiovascular dynamics and block the increase in stress-responsive hormones that normally occur with surgical stimulation. Animal and patient studies were successful, and the technique called analgesic-anesthesia was reported at the World Congress of Anesthesiology in Mexico City in 1976.

The offer to use fentanyl in the healthcare system of the United States of America was initially not met with the expected response due to concerns about the possible abuse of the substance in the drug scene. It was not until 1968 that fentanyl mixed with droperidol in a ratio of 50:1 droperidol to fentanyl was approved by the U.S. Food and Drug Administration (FDA) for use in clinical anesthesiology under the name Innovar. In other countries, it was used under the name Thalamonal. Six years later, fentanyl was also used alone, in 1 mL ampoules containing 50 μg of the active substance [4].

Today, it is widely used for preoperative analgesia, general anesthesia, anesthesia adjunct, regional anesthesia adjunct, postoperative pain control, and moderate to severe acute pain (off-label). Fentanyl must be titrated with increased caution and care for patients with lung disease, impaired liver or kidney function, alcohol dependence, or hypothyroidism [5].

2. Pharmacochemical properties

Fentanyl is rapidly distributed with sequestration in fat and binds to human plasma proteins. It is metabolized mainly in the liver and is excreted by the kidneys.

The elimination half-life ranges from 6 to 32 h. With intravenous administration, it works almost immediately, with intramuscular administration it takes about 7–8 min. The maximum effect that the drug achieves is observed in 5–15 min after intravenous injection. Analgesic effect with intramuscular administration is 1–2 h. It has a faster onset and shorter duration of action than morphine. The pharmacokinetics of fentanyl is described as a three-compartment model with a distribution time of 1.7 min, a redistribution of 13 min, and a terminal elimination half-life of 219 min. The volume of distribution is 4 L/kg.

Fentanyl belongs to the strong opioids; it is an agonist of μ-opioid receptors. Fentanyl acts preferentially on μ receptors. All fentanyl-type compounds (a series of 4-anilidopiperidines) are highly μ-selective but could also form affinity for δ- and κ-opiate receptors.

It is highly lipophilic, undergoes first-pass metabolism by the liver, is absorbed very quickly through the oral mucosa, and more slowly through the classic gastrointestinal route. Its administration in oral dosage forms is practically impossible. For this reason, it is only available for parenteral application in anesthesiology and intensive care. Transdermal fentanyl systems have been successfully used in algesiology to address chronic pain in oncology patients.

Among physicians and other professionals, the use of fentanyl opioids for pain relief is highly preferred mainly due to their favorable pharmacochemical properties. Fentanyl maintains cardiac stability and, in certain doses, reduces stress-related hormonal changes. From a number of fentanyl derivatives, it is fentanyl, alfentanil, remifentanil, and sufentanil in the form of salts (fentanyl dihydrogen citrate, alfentanil hydrochloride, remifentanil hydrochloride, and sufentanil dihydrogen citrate) that are allowed to be used in human medicine.

Pain treatment is always started with the lowest possible dose of opioid, taking into account the adverse effects of the substance and the patient's health. The value of the therapeutic index, which provides information on the relative safety of the drug, is essential for the choice of opioids in the treatment of pain. It is given by the ratio between the dose that is toxic for the 50% of the population and effective for the 50% of the population. TI = TD50/ED50. The higher the TI, the greater the relative safety of the drug [6].

The recommended serum concentration for analgesia is 1–2 ng/mL and for anesthesia 10–20 ng/mL. Blood concentrations of approximately 7 ng/mL or higher have been associated with fatal outcomes when multiple agents are involved. During the past decades, a number of studies have been conducted comparing doses for anesthesia of patients, for example, anesthesia was maintained with infusions of propofol (50–100 μg/kg/min) and either remifentanil (0.2 μg/kg/min), alfentanil (20 μg/kg/h), or fentanyl (2 μg/kg/h) [7].

When comparing the effects of alfentanil and remifentanil, it was found that both drugs are pharmacokinetically similar, but the central clearance of remifentanil is significantly higher. Population pharmacokinetic parameters of remifentanil include CLc of 2.9 L/min, corresponding parameters for alfentanil are 0.36 L/min. Pharmacodynamically, the drugs are similar, but remifentanil is 19 times more potent than alfentanil, with an effective concentration for 50% maximal effect of 19.9 ng/mL versus 375.9 ng/mL for alfentanil [8, 9].

In pediatric patients, fentanyl and remifentanil were experimentally administered intraoperatively in doses of 0.2 μg/kg/min remifentanil and 2 μg/kg during induction of anesthesia [10, 11].

Like other opioids, fentanyl and its derivatives are characterized by adverse effects, including nausea and vomiting, fatigue, headache, dizziness, constipation, miosis, anemia, bradycardia, and respiratory depression. After stopping use, withdrawal symptoms characteristic of opioids (sweating, anxiety, diarrhea, bone pain, abdominal cramps, and chills) may appear. Serious health problems are reported when fentanyl is mixed with heroin, cocaine, alcohol, and other central nervous system depressants, such as benzodiazepines. Based on pooled safety data from these clinical trials, the most commonly reported adverse reactions were nausea (35.7%), vomiting (23.2%), constipation (23.1%), somnolence (15.0%), dizziness (13, 1%), and headache (11.8%). All opioids of the fentanyl series can only be administered under conditions where monitoring and support of respiratory and cardiovascular functions is fully ensured [12, 13].

Many experiments on animals are continuously carried out to help explain the effects of fentanyl on the human body. For instance, it was found that in mice the onset of respiratory depression occurs 70 times faster after the administration of fentanyl compared to morphine [14].

In human medicine, fentanyl is administered to patients in several forms, taking into account whether the parenteral route is useful for the patient—penetration of the active substance through the skin, transmucosal and nasal (mucosal) route (transmucosal and nasal administration), and intravenous administration or sublingual administration.

A common application form before performing a surgical procedure is the intravenous administration of a drug solution. Fentanyl Dihydrogen citrate 0.0785 mg/ml, which corresponds to Fentanyl 0.050 mg/ml, is usually administered. The dose of fentanyl is determined individually according to age, body weight, physical condition, pathological conditions, and current treatment, as well as the type of surgery and the type of anesthesia. The dosage regimens listed below are recommended. For neuroleptic analgesia in adults, the usual starting dose is 50–100 μg (0.7–1.4 μg/kg) fentanyl, administered slowly intravenously in combination with neuroleptics (preferably with droperidol). If a second dose of 50–100 μg (0.7–1.4 μg/kg) is required, fentanyl can be administered 30–45 min after the initial dose.

For neuroleptic anesthesia under conditions of controlled pulmonary ventilation in adults, an initial dose of 200–600 μg (2.8–8.4 μg/kg) of fentanyl is generally administered, slowly intravenously in combination with neuroleptics (preferably with droperidol). The dose depends on the duration and severity of the surgical procedure and on the treatment used for general anesthesia. To prolong anesthesia, additional doses of 50–100 μg (0.7–1.4 μg/kg) of fentanyl can be given every 30–45 min. The time intervals and size of further doses are adjusted depending on the course of the medical procedure. For pediatric patients, doses are adapted to the age and condition of the child. In children from 2 to 12 years of age, a single analgesic dose of 1–3 μg of fentanyl/kg of body weight is administered, for example., in combination with inhalation anesthetics. 1.25 μg/kg fentanyl may be administered to maintain analgesia during general anesthesia, depending on the course of the operation. Higher doses of fentanyl are required in patients chronically treated with opioids or with a known history of opioid overdose [15].

Fentanyl is usually administered in preoperative analgesia in a dose of 50–100 μg intravenously 30–60 min before surgery, in general anesthesia 20–50 μg/kg intravenously, and in supplementary anesthesia 2–50 μg per dose intravenously. For elderly patients, 65 years and older, a lower dose is recommended. In high-risk patients undergoing a demanding surgical procedure, it is advisable to supplement the anesthesia with oxygen and increase the dose of fentanyl to 150 μg/kg. For postoperative pain control, administration of 50–100 μg every 1–2 h as needed is recommended [16].

One form of fentanyl use through the skin is transdermal application.

The transdermal therapeutic system (TTS) was developed as an adequate substitute for oral or parenteral drug administration. It is therapeutically usable in case of need for a longer duration of effect of the substance for patients with chronic pain and to prevent possible adverse consequences of treatment occurring in the case of other forms of administration. The advantage is the possibility of setting a balanced level of the opioid acting on the organism, without exposing the patient's gastrointestinal tract to discomfort [17, 18]. Transdermal fentanyl patches are manufactured, containing a reservoir with the active substance, adjusted to deliver the required amount of substance over the course of 3 days. A base dose is incorporated into the adhesive layer to saturate certain binding sites in the skin and to accelerate the achievement of steady-state blood levels. Fentanyl patches are typically designed by the manufacturer to release approximately 12.5, 25, 50, 75 and 100 μg of fentanyl per hour into the systemic circulation, depending on the patient's medical condition. After 72 h, the patch should be removed and a new one applied to a different location. TTS has an important place in therapy, especially to prevent repeated oral doses, or when oral therapy is evaluated as ineffective or intolerable. The predecessor of fentanyl patches was the successful and verified administration of the substance scopolamine during the 1980s [19].

Subsequently, a patch containing fentanyl (called Duragesic) was created, for which FDA and European regulatory approval was later obtained (**Figure 1**) [20].

Studies were conducted in patients with acute postoperative pain, previously untreated with opioids, but it caused too much respiratory depression. When it was later evaluated in opioid-tolerant patients with chronic cancer-induced pain in the late 1980s and early 1990s, the patch was shown to be useful for the ability to maintain a steady blood level of fentanyl for 2–3 days and was approved by the FDA and European regulatory authorities [21]. Despite the initial doubts of Dr. Janssen, the transdermal opioid was recognized as a successful drug for chronic pain in cancer patients [4]. Fentanyl Orion, for example, is available on the market to manage severe chronic pain, the properties of which are listed in **Table 1**.

The dosage is always individual and is based on the previous administration of opioid analgesics, taking into account the severity of the disease, the patient's current

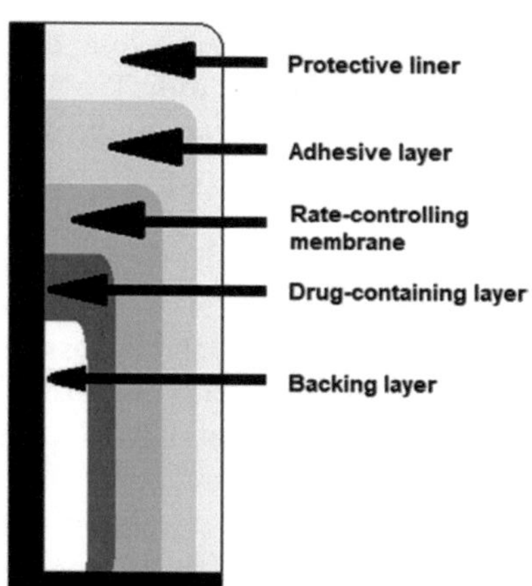

Figure 1.
Diagram of a transdermal patch with an active substance.

Designation of patch type	12.5	25	50	75	100
Active substance content (mg)	2.55	5.1	10.2	15.3	20.4
Patch area (cm^2)	4.25	8.5	17.0	25.5	34.0
Fentanyl release rate (μg/h)	12.5	25.0	50.0	75.0	100.0

Table 1.
Patch properties.

state of health, the possible development of tolerance, the possibility of a collision due to other administered drugs, or the onset of contraindications [22].

The danger of overdose lies mainly in the difference in the content of the active substance in the patch, and especially in the case of patches already used by the patient, the residual concentration of the extracted fentanyl is completely unknown to the user. In addition to fatal overdose, users are at risk of various ischemic injuries, limb amputation, thrombophlebitis, and severe skin ulcers. Other serious consequences include endocarditis, septic embolism, and osteomyelitis [23].

A suitable method for fast, safe, and easy application of fentanyl is transmucosal administration, whether in oral, buccal, or sublingual form, because lipophilic drugs, such as fentanyl, are easily and quickly absorbed by the mucous membrane [24]. With the development of pain treatment, new routes of fentanyl administration are being developed, which are intended for the treatment of PB: orotransmucosal systems (lollipops, sublingual tablets) and intranasal spray [25, 26], and there are also mentions of the possibility of transpulmonary administration of fentanyl by inhalation [27]. The principle of the new medicinal form of fentanyl intended for buccal application (FBT—fentanyl buccal tablet) is a technology using an effervescent reaction that increases the speed and extent of absorption of the oral mucosa [28].

The first mucosal application method was an OTFC (oral transmucosal fentanyl citrate) lollipop [29] called Oralet. Due to the lack of Oralet's clinical success, Actic was later produced, intended for patients with oncological diseases already on opioid treatment [4]. It has been used for breakthrough pain for more than a decade and is particularly suitable for pediatric patients. Buccal [30] or sublingual [31] application is made possible by a fast-dissolving tablet, where fentanyl is bound to a carrier that adheres to the mucosa and can act for a sufficiently long time. The onset is very fast, and the maximum effect is achieved within 30 min. The effect lasts up to 240 min. From the point of view of patient comfort (meaning the elimination of fear and anxiety), this form of fentanyl administration appears to be very advantageous. Application by the transmucosal route has its origin in an experiment with the sedation of larger animals in the state of Utah with carfentanil. This form of administration has been found to have the advantage of a simple application that does not stress the patient. Studies on monkeys have shown that it is possible to ensure the comfort of animals by, for instance, giving a sugar cube with a sedative. After a few minutes, the animals were either completely anesthetized or allowed to be handled by the veterinarian, depending on the size of the dose.

With an overdose of fentanyl and its derivatives, respiratory depression is especially dangerous, and respiratory assistance is the priority in such cases. The antidote given in overdose is a strong opioid antagonist—naloxone (also known as naltrexone, nalmefene, and so forth), which blocks μ-receptors and can, therefore, be used both in overdoses with fentanyl, heroin, and other new synthetic opioids [32, 33].

3. Chemical properties of fentanyl

The chemical structure of fentanyl, a substance with the chemical name *N*-(1-phenethyl-4-piperidyl) propionamide and the formula $C_{22}H_{28}N_2O$, is a monocarboxylic acid amide. It contains a relatively simple skeleton with four important parts, namely the amide group, aniline, piperidine ring, and alkyl chain linked to s tertiary nitrogen (**Figure 2**).

It was patented in 1965 under the number U.S. Pat. No. 3,164,600 ('600) [34, 35]. The synthesis consisted of several parts, namely:

i. refluxing mixture of 1-benzyl-4-piperidone, aniline, toluene, and 4 toluene-sulfonic acid for 15 h to produce *N*-(1-benzyl-4-piperydylidene)aniline,

ii. reducing *N*-(1-benzyl-4-piperydylidene)aniline is obtained using lithium aluminum hydride in anhydrous ether to 1-benzyl-4-anilinopiperidine in nitrogen atmosphere, then

iii. alkalizing by refluxing with propionic anhydride for 7 h to give *N*-(1-benzyl-4-piperydylidene)propionanilide,

iv. subjecting to debenzylation by employing hydrogenation over palladium on charcoal catalyst in ethanol to get *N*-(4-piperidyl)propionanilide, and finally

v. treating a mixture of *N*-(4-piperidyl)propionanilide, sodium carbonate, and potassium iodide in hexone with the solution of β phenethylchloride in 4-methyl-2-pentanone and refluxed for 27 h to obtain fentanyl.

Due to the time-consuming nature of the synthesis, the relatively low yield, and the current requirements for environmental quality, it underwent several modifications in later years [36, 37]. The basic skeletal structure of fentanyl can be advantageously modified at fourmolecule positions [38, 39].

Some selected properties of fentanyl are listed in **Table 2**.

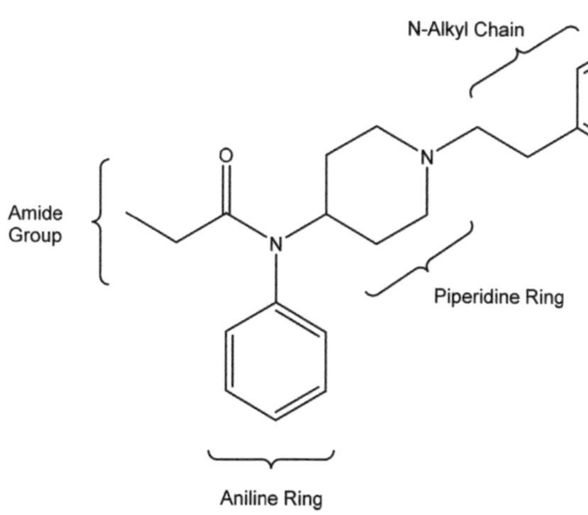

Figure 2.
Structure of fentanyl.

Chemical properties of fentanyl	
Appearance	White crystals or powder
Molar mass [g/mol]	336.5
Melting point [°C]	85.2
Water solubility [mg/L]	200 (25 °C)
pK_a value	8.4
Number of hydrogen bond donors	0
Number of hydrogen bond donors	6
Heavy atom count (no hydrogen)	25

Table 2.
Chemical properties of fentanyl [40].

4. Fentanyl analogues

Janssen's first synthesis of fentanyl, which is based on *N*-benzyl-4-piperidone, has been effectively modified several times over the years. Expansion and contraction of the piperidine ring were performed, and a series of conformationally restricted fentanyl analogs were stereochemically characterized, methyl substituents and others, for example, 4-phenyl group were inserted into various positions of the fentanyl molecule, the phenyl ring was replaced by heteroaromatic thienyls or tetrazolyl rings, and a number of other changes were performed. Thus, hundreds of new fentanyl derivatives were created.

A relationship between the structure of substances and their activity of fentanyl compounds exists. Compounds with a 4-*N*-anilinopiperidine group (except *N*-methyl derivatives) are known to show high affinity for μ-receptors. High activity and affinity to μ-receptors are also caused by the methyl substitution at the third position of the piperidine ring and the presence of a 4-carboxymethyl or 4-methoxymethyl substituent. It was also found that methyl substitution at the second position of the piperidine ring does not cause a significant change in activity. However, many questions remain unanswered such as the fact that fentanyl, sufentanil, methylfentanyl, and lofentanil are more effective than could be expected based on the obtained binding values [2, 41].

In addition to fentanyl, its derivatives alfentanil, remifentanil, and sufentanil are permitted for use in the healthcare sector, sufentanil, and carfentanil are used in veterinary practice:

Alfentanil, ($C_{21}H_{32}N_6O_3$), a piperidine with a 2-(4-ethyl-5-oxo-4,5-dihydro-1*H*-tetrazol-1-yl)ethyl group in position 1, as well as *N*-phenylpropanamido- and methoxymethyl groups in position 4 [42]. It is suitable for neuroleptanalgesia in ambulatory surgery with shorter medical procedure time. It accumulates in tissues less than fentanyl and has more favorable pharmacokinetic properties. It was synthesized in the laboratories of Janssen Pharmaceutica in 1976, and in the pharmaceutical industry, it is referred to as Alfenta®, Rapifen [43]. Intravenous administration is common. However, other routes of alfentanil administration, including epidural (injection into the epidural space), intrathecal (injection into the spinal canal or subarachnoid space), transdermal (through the skin), and intranasal, have demonstrated the expected and desired efficacy. Potential adverse effects are similar to those of other opioids, but the observed specificity of alfentanil compared to other derivatives is the reduction of pressure and the induction of chest wall stiffness [44, 45]. The risk or severity of adverse effects may increase if alfentanil is combined, for instance, with 1,2-benzodiazepine [46].

Remifentanil, methyl 1-(3-methoxy-3-oxopropyl)-4-(*N*-propanoylanilino)piperidine-4-carboxylate, substance with general formula $C_{20}H_{28}N_2O_5$, is a white, water-soluble powder, known in the field of pharmacy under the former name GI-87084B [47]. Due to the absence of a chiral center, it exists in only one form. It contains a piperidinecarboxylate ester in its molecule, which is methylpiperidine-4-carboxylate, in which the hydrogen bound to the nitrogen is substituted by a 3-methoxy-3-oxopropyl group. The hydrogen at position 4 is substituted by the nitrogen of *N*-propanoylaniline.

It is split by nonspecific esterases in plasma and tissues. In healthcare, it is used in the form of hydrochloride. It is administered to adult patients as an intravenous infusion in doses ranging from 0.1 to 0.5 (μg/kg)/min [48]. In the blood, it is relatively quickly inactivated by esterases into inactive metabolites; therefore, it has a very short effect and good controllability duration of action. The substance is used for short-term analgesia during ambulatory procedures, but it has almost zero use in the treatment of chronic pain. Concomitant medication is carried out with propofol and isoflurane [49, 50].

Sufentanil, an anilide synthesized by formal condensation of the arylamino group of 4-(methoxymethyl)-*N*-phenyl-1-[2-(2-thienyl)ethyl]piperidin-4-amine with propanoic acid [51], is a white or off-white powder previously also known under the name R 3073, with the general formula $C_{22}H_{30}N_2O_2S$. It is practically insoluble in water; however, it is easily soluble in methanol and ethanol (96%). It is known under the brand names Sufenta® and Sufenta Forte. It has up to 10x greater analgesic effect than fentanyl, 30× higher affinity for opioid receptors [52], and is extremely fat soluble, allowing rapid penetration into the central nervous system. The duration of its effect is approximately 10–25 min. In combination with propofol, it creates acceptable conditions for incubating the patient without administering a muscle relaxant. The advantage over fentanyl is a shorter biological half-life. Its high therapeutic index of 25,000 and minimal respiratory depression predetermine this substance for use in the medical environment. Experimental work comparing, for example, sublingual sufentanil in an administered amount of 30 μg and fentanyl in an amount of 50 μg did not confirm a significant difference in analgesic assistance [53–55].

Carfentanil is the most powerful opioid known. Its systematic name is methyl 1-(2-phenylethyl)-4-[phenyl(propanoyl)amino]piperidine-4-carboxylate), and the general formula is $C_{24}H_{30}N_2O_3$. Carfentanil is a monocarboxylic acid amide formed by the formal condensation of the arylamino group methyl-4-anilino-1-(2-phenylethyl) of piperidine-4-carboxylate with propanoic acid [56]. It is an analgesic with an approximately 10,000 times stronger analgesic effect compared to morphine. It was first synthesized in 1974 (trademark Wildnil®) and was approved for use as an intramuscular tranquilizer for large animals (rhinoceros, bears, and elephants) in 1986. However, other methods of application, such as intravenous, oral, and transmucosal, are also approved. The usual dosage for a 6-ton elephant is 10 mg intravenously. For human purposes, the use of carfentanil is not allowed. The estimated threshold dose in humans is 1–2 μg, and the effective dose 8–15 μg/kg administered intramuscularly [57, 58].

Lofentanil, the most effective known fentanyl derivative to date, was created by modifying the central fentanyl piperidine ring (similar to e.g., carfentanil), which induces significant analgesia lasting up to 8–12 h. It has been clinically tested during epidural application, but the disadvantage is the resulting severe respiratory depression and problems in antagonizing its effect with the classic opioid antagonist—naloxone [52]. Due to steric hindrances caused by its structure and extremely high toxicity, it is used only for experimental studies of opiate receptors and is not allowed in human or veterinary practice [59, 60] as it induces anesthesia already at a dose of 0.025 g/kg of body weight, while, for instance, the expected lethal dose of the nerve agent labeled VX, *O*-ethyl-*S*-(2-diisopropylaminoethyl)methylphosphonothiolate, is 100 times higher [61].

Acryloylfentanyl, (sometimes written as acrylfentanyl), is a derivative of fentanyl whose detection in forensic analysis is difficult due to the fact that it differs from the fentanyl molecule only by the presence of an extra double bond. Acryloylfentanyl differs from fentanyl in the double bond present in the 2-position of the propane attached to the *N*-phenyl moiety and is, therefore, an unsaturated analog of fentanyl. Like many other derivatives, it contains one basic nitrogen atom in the piperidine ring, so it can easily form salts with organic or inorganic acids. The synthesis and antinociceptive activity of acryloylfentanyl was first described in 1981. It is also known by the names acryloyl-F, Acr-F, and ACF. It shows about 170 times stronger effect compared to morphine but weaker effect compared to fentanyl [62, 63].

Other synthetic "nonmedical" opioids that were not included among pharmaceutical products are acetylfentanyl, butyrfentanyl, furanylfentanyl, ocfentanil, and other fentanyl derivatives [64].

5. Abuse of fentanyl-series opioids

The abuse of fentanyl and its derivatives by drug addicts is a worldwide problem. Although the amount of new synthetic opioids seized by the police is lower in percentage compared to substances such as cocaine, cannabinoids, cathinones, and others, it is necessary to be aware of their potency. High efficiency significantly increases the level of danger to the health of individuals and society. The substances of the fentanyl series are considered a relatively attractive and profitable commodity for organized crime. They are offered directly *via* the Internet, the so-called darknet, or as counterfeit drugs or mixtures with other substances. The opioids are administered by known application routes, using tablets, nasal spray, or injection. The danger of the illegal market for users lies primarily in the fact that it is not certain whether the declared content of the active ingredient corresponds to reality, such as in the case of tablets [64], as shown in the picture (**Figure 3**).

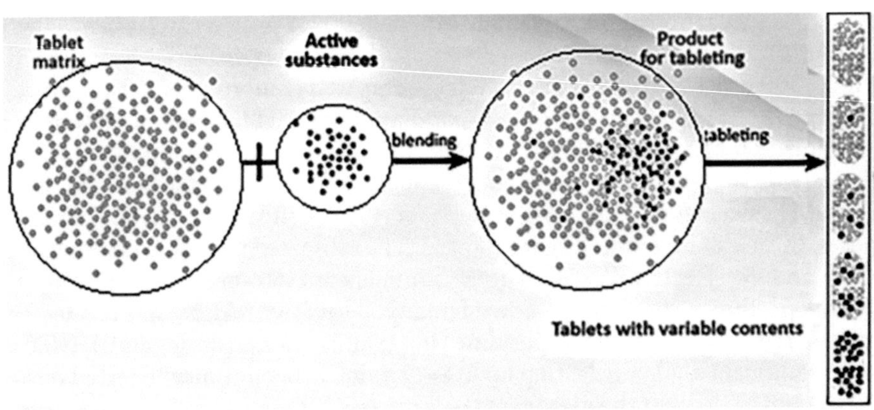

Figure 3.
Different distribution of the active substance in illegally produced tablets [64].

Drug addicts obtain some opioids not only from illegal laboratories but also from legal supplies of medicinal products, such as transdermal patches. The users extract fentanyl from the patches and inject it intravenously without maintaining sterile conditions, chew the patches, apply a large number of patches to the skin, inhale the smoke from a heated patch, and so forth [65].

Opioids continue to lead the way in overdose deaths. There have been over 91,000 overdose deaths in North America, a number greatly increased by fentanyl, with estimates for 2021 of over 107,000 deaths. According to the 2022 data from forensic toxicologists in Canada, up to 86% of deaths are caused by the illegal ingestion of fentanyl or its derivatives. The cause is the high toxicity of illicit drugs, the detected concentrations exceed 50 μg/L. Carfentanil was identified in 126 deaths in 2022 [66, 67]. On the European continent, the situation with opioid consumption is less problematic compared to the United States. Higher consumption and reports of overdose deaths are reported from the United Kingdom and Scotland [68, 69].

On March 31, 1961, the single convention on narcotic drugs was negotiated in New York, which aimed to curb drug abuse through coordinated action at the international level. The convention establishes a system of international control of psychotropic substances based on the likelihood of abuse and on the other hand according to their therapeutic index. All EU member states are parties to the convention on narcotic drugs and the convention on psychotropic substances. There is interagency cooperation and coordination of efforts in addressing and countering the world drug problem. The activities of the United Nations Office on Drugs and Crime (UNODC) are known, whose mission is to contribute to global security by making the world safer from drugs, crime, and terrorism.

In view of the critical global drug abuse situation, the UNODC early warning board (EWA) was established in 2013 to monitor, analyze, and report on trends in the consumption and abuse of new psychoactive substances. It stores the obtained data and provides technical assistance to member states. EWA is managed by the UNODC global synthetics monitoring: Analyses, Reporting, and Trends (SMART) program.

Dangerous synthetic fentanyl-type psychoactive substances that are frequently reported from forensic laboratories or police seizures include 4-methoxybutyrfentanyl, acryloylfentanyl, butyrfentanyl, despropionylfentanyl, despropionyl-2-fluorofentanyl, furanylfentanyl, para-fluoroisobutyrfentanyl, valerylfentanyl, (iso)butyrfentanyl, (iso)butyr-F-fentanyl *N*-benzyl analog, acetylfentanyl (controlled under Schedule I of the 1961 Single Convention on Narcotic Drugs), ocfentanil, and beta-hydroxythiofentanyl [70].

Acetylfentanyl, for example, is about 16 times more potent than morphine, and the therapeutic index is relatively low, which increases the risk of fatal overdose. It appears on the illegal market in the USA, Europe, Japan, China, and Australia as a substitute for fentanyl or heroin. Sometimes, he is called sometimes being called the "first apostle of extinction". Police seizures of this substance are reported from the USA, some European countries, and China [71].

Butyrylfentanyl, such as acetylfentanyl and other fentanyl opioids, poses a potential overdose risk without legitimate clinical use despite being about times less potent than fentanyl. Dozens of deaths linked to butyrylfentanyl abuse have been reported. It is also legislatively controlled [72].

Another fentanyl analog, 4-fluorobutyrylfentanyl, is often available mixed with heroin and is the cause of many deaths [73].

The report of the International Narcotics Control Board (Report of the International Narcotics Control Board) shows that attention must also be paid to the so-called precursors in the synthesis of fentanyl. The substance 4-anilidopiperidine (4-AP) is a substitution chemical for *N*-phenethyl-4-piperidone (NPP) for the synthesis of 4-anilino-*N*-phenethylpiperidine (ANPP), which itself was an immediate precursor for the production of fentanyl and some of its analogs. NPP and ANPP were included in Schedule I of the 1988 convention in 2017 [74, 75].

The properties and risks of addictive substances are continuously assessed by the Scientific Committee of the European Monitoring Center for Drugs and Drug Addiction, and many are legislatively controlled at international level under the Single Convention on Narcotic Drugs of 1961 [76].

6. Instrumental methods of detecting the presence of fentanyl

Qualitative and quantitative analyzes of opioids, including fentanyl, are performed in biological materials—urine, blood, plasma, and hair. Postmortem concentrations of fentanyl opioids detected in the blood of victims are extremely low in the range of picograms per milliliter (pg/mL), which in a certain way presents a challenge for forensic laboratories dealing with analyzes of these substances. Both simple orientation methods and sophisticated instrumentation are used to detect their presence. Tests based on the principle of immunochemical methods, often originally developed to control biological samples, are used for rapid field testing. The indicated cut-off concentrations are 200 ng/mL [77, 78].

Indicative information about fentalogs can also be obtained by the proven method of thin-layer chromatography, where the emphasis is primarily on simplicity and financial simplicity while maintaining maximum reproducibility of results. In this method, attention is focused on the choice of suitable chromatographic systems in combination with various detection reagents [79].

A relatively simple, fast, and cheap method, used primarily to determine the amount of the substance of interest, is the analysis of extraction spectrometry in the visible radiation range. The base of the method is that the amine nitrogen present in the fentalogs molecule provides ion pairs with acid dyes, which can then be extracted with nonpolar solvents and subjected to measurements on proven single-beam or double-beam spectrometers [80].

The presence of fentanyl and its derivatives, or other drugs, can also be determined using the electrochemical-surface enhanced Raman spectroscopy (EC-SERS) method. Detection limits for fentanyl compounds were found to be in the low nanogram per milliliter range, with the most sensitive compound detected at 10 ng/mL. This analysis was successful even when the sample contained 5–1% fentanyl [81, 82]. The method is highly selective for the analysis of fentanyl in the presence of some interfering compounds, including cocaine, heroin, and methamphetamine. It represents a powerful application for screening seized drugs in the laboratory and at the crime scene.

Known methods, often used to determine fentanyl and its derivatives, are electroanalytical methods such as voltammetry, potentiometry, and electrochemiluminescence [83].

Accurate identification of opioids can be performed with analytical systems with high separation capability, such as gas or liquid chromatography, which is usually coupled with mass spectrometry [84].

Current modern devices stand out for their high scanning speed, minimal requirements for the amount of the controlled substance, programmable temperature and other technical advantages that enable quick and accurate obtaining of the desired result. Distinction of structural isomers is provided, for instance, by HPLC-DOD, LC-MS/MS, or LC-QToF-MS with quadrupole and others [85, 86].

From this analysis, it emerges that the gold standard for the identification and quantification of 4-anilinopiperidines is LC-MS/MS, coupled with liquid-liquid or solid-phase extraction [87].

A very sensitive LC-MS/MS method for the multiplex detection of analogs and their metabolites in blood, namely for fentanyl, norfentanyl, furanylfentanyl, furanylnorfentanyl, butyrylnorfentanyl, acetylfentanyl, alfentanil, acryloylfentanyl, remifentanil, sufentanil, *p*-methoxyfentanyl, carfentanil, (±)-*cis*-3-methylfentanyl, butyrylfentanyl, isobutyrylfentanyl, valerylfentanyl, and others, was successfully applied with results of concentrations in the range of 0.1–0.5 ng/mL [88].

7. Fentanyl usage by armed forces

The use of substances that affect the central nervous system was originally intended for the medical field. However, their importance has also extended to the military sphere, where they can be used, for instance, in managing critical situations.

Fentanyl, as an interesting type of opioid, became more widely known to the lay public mainly after the incident in Moscow in 2002 when the army of the Russian federation used a mixture of fentanyl derivatives in the form of an aerosol to rescue hostages in the Dubrovka theater occupied by Chechen separatists as part of an anti-terrorist operation. In 2012, Porton Down laboratory workers published information on the composition of the aerosol used in Moscow after analyzing samples of clothing and urine from people in the Moscow theater; it was a mixture of remifentanil and carfentanil, still illegal in human medicine and very potent [89]. As a potential chemical incapacitating agent, fentanyl was already investigated in the 1970s by the Soviet KGB under the name Kolokol-1 [90].

The effects of incapacitating chemical substances raise questions about their legitimate use in armed conflicts, hostage-taking crises, maintaining public order, or peacekeeping missions. Due to the need for new strategies that could help reduce the number of deaths and injuries, this issue has been debated by individual states for decades [91–93].

Author details

Romana Jelínková
NBC Defence Institute Vyskov, University of Defence, Brno, Czech Republic

*Address all correspondence to: romana.jelinkova@unob.cz

IntechOpen

© 2024 The Author(s). Licensee IntechOpen. This chapter is distributed under the terms of the Creative Commons Attribution License (http://creativecommons.org/licenses/by/3.0), which permits unrestricted use, distribution, and reproduction in any medium, provided the original work is properly cited.

References

[1] Lüllmann H, Mohr K, Welhing M. Farmakologie a toxikologie. 2nd ed. Praha: Grada Publishing; 2004. ISBN 80-247-0836-1

[2] Vardanyan RS, Hruby VJ. Fentanyl-related compounds and derivatives: Current status and future prospects for pharmaceutical applications. Future Medicinal Chemistry. 2014;**6**(4):385-412. DOI: 10.4155/fmc.13.215

[3] Fentanyl Citrate Injection, USP. Reference ID: 3336008 [Internet]. 2013. Available from: https://www.accessdata.fda.gov/drugsatfda_docs/label/2013/016619s034lbl.pdf [Accessed: May 19, 2023]

[4] Stanley TH. The fentanyl story. The Journal of Pain. 2014;**15**(12):1215-1226. DOI: 10.1016/j.jpain.2014.08.010

[5] Kawanaka R, Sakuma S, Kokubun H, et al. Effects of intraoperative opioid administration on postoperative pain and pain threshold: A randomized controlled study. Journal of Clinical Medicine. 2022;**11**(19):5587. DOI: 10.3390/jcm11195587

[6] Gable R. Comparison of acute lethal toxicity of commonly abused psychoactive substances. Addiction (Abingdon, England). 2004;**99**:686-696. DOI: 10.1111/j.1360-0443.2004.00744.x

[7] Coles PJ et al. Propofol anesthesia for craniotomy: A double-blind comparison of remifentanil, alfentanil, and fentanyl. Journal of Neurosurgical Anesthesiology. 2000;**12**(1):15-20. DOI: 10.1097/00008506-200001000-00004

[8] Egan TD, Minto CF, Hermann DJ, Barr J, Muir KT, Shafer SL. Remifentanil versus alfentanil: Comparative pharmacokinetics and pharmacodynamics in healthy adult male volunteers. Anesthesiology. 1996;**84**(4):821-833. DOI: 10.1097/00000542-199604000-00009. Erratum in: Anesthesiology 1996;85(3):695

[9] Hughes LM, Irwin MG, Nestor CC. Alternatives to remifentanil for the analgesic component of total intravenous anaesthesia: A narrative review. Anaesthesia. 2023;**78**(5):620-625. DOI: 10.1111/anae.15952

[10] Baek J, Park SJ, Kim JO, et al. The effects of remifentanil and fentanyl on emergence agitation in pediatric strabismus surgery. Children (Basel). 2022;**24**(5):606. DOI: 10.3390/children9050606

[11] Choi EK, Lee S, Kim WJ, Park SJ. Effects of remifentanil maintenance during recovery on emergence delirium in children with sevoflurane anesthesia. Paediatric Anaesthesia. 2018;**28**(8):739-744. DOI: 10.1111/pan.13446

[12] Boysen PG, Patel JH, King AN. Brief history of opioids in perioperative and periprocedural medicine to inform the future. Ochsner Journal. 2023;**23**(1):43-49. DOI: 10.31486/toj.22.0065

[13] State Institute for Drug Control [Internet]. 2011. Available from: https://www.sukl.cz/download/spc/SPC31591.pdf [Accessed: May 20, 2021]

[14] Hill R, Santhakumar R, Dewey W, Kelly E, Henderson G. Fentanyl depression of respiration: Comparison with heroin and morphine. British Journal of Pharmacology. 2020;**177**:254-265. DOI: 10.1111/bph.14860

[15] FENTANYL TORREX 50 μg/ml [Internet]. 2011. Available from: https://www.sukl.cz/download/pil/PI20569.pdf [Accessed: May 14, 2023]

[16] Carlos FR-M, Bistas KG, Lopez-Ojeda W. Fentanyl [Internet]. 2023. Available from: https://www.ncbi.nlm.nih.gov/books/NBK459275/ [Accessed: June 12, 2023]

[17] Eissenberg E, McNicol ED, Carr DB. Efficacy of mi-opioi agonist in treatment of evoked neuropathic pain: Systematic review of randomized controlled trials. European Journal of Pain. 2006;**10**(8):667-676. DOI: 10.1016/j.ejpain.2005.10.007

[18] Moore KT et al. Bioequivalence and safety of a novel fentanyl transdermal matrix system compared with a transdermal reservoir system. Journal of Opioid Management. 2011;**7**(2):99-107. DOI: 10.5055/jom.2011.0052

[19] Zohar N, Shupak A, Gordon CR. Transdermal scopolamine for prevention of motion sickness: Clinical pharmacokinetics and therapeutic applications. Clinical Pharmacokinetics. 2006;**45**(6):543-566. DOI: 10.2165/00003088-200645060-00001

[20] Kress HG, Boss H, Delvin T, et al. Transdermal fentanyl matrix patches Matrifen® and Durogesic® DTrans® are bioequivalent. European Journal of Pharmaceutics and Biopharmaceutics. 2010;**75**(2):225-231. DOI: /10.1016/j.ejpb.2010.02.005

[21] Stanley TH. Anesthesia for the 21st century. Proceedings (Baylor University. Medical Center). 2000;**13**(1):7-10. DOI: 10.1080/08998280.2000.11927635

[22] Chen J, Zou X, Hu B, et al. Effect of different doses of esketamine compared with fentanyl combined with propofol on hypotension in patients undergoing painless abortion surgery: A prospective, randomized, double-blind controlled clinical trial. BMC Anesthesiology. 2022;**22**:305. DOI: 10.1186/s12871-022-01848-6

[23] The Dangers of Abusing Fentanyl Patches. Drug & Alcohol Rehab Centers [Internet]. 2019. Available from: https://americanaddictioncenters.org/fentanyl-treatment/dangers-of-abuse [Accessed: March 26, 2020]

[24] Payne R, Coluzzi P, Hart L, et al. Longterm safety of oral transmucosal fentanyl citrate for breakthrough cancer pain. Journal of Pain Management. 2001;**22**:575-583. DOI: 10.1016/s0885-3924(01)00306-2

[25] Heshmati F, Noroozinia H, Abbasivash R, et al. Intranasal sufentanil for postoperative pain control in lower abdominal pediatric surgery. IJPT. 2006;**5**:131-133

[26] Corrigan M, Wilson SS, Hampto J. Safety and efficacy of intranasally administered medications in the emergency department and prehospital settings. American Journal of Health-System Pharmacy. 2015;**72**:1544-1554. DOI: 10.2146/ajhp140630

[27] Bevans T, Deering-Rice C, Stockmann C, et al. Inhaled remifentanil in rodents. Anesthesia and Analgesia. 2016;**122**:1831-1838. DOI: 10.1213/ANE.0000000000001228

[28] Nosková V. Fentanyl v bukální formě – nové řešení průlomové bolesti [Internet]. 2010. Available from: https://www.remedia.cz/rubriky/klinicka-farmakologie-a-farmacie/fentanyl-v-bukalni-forme-nove-reseni-prulomove-bolesti-3457/ [Accessed: January 15, 2023]. In Czech Language

[29] Singh RB, Choubey S, Mehra R. Efficacy of oral transmucosal fentanyl citrate for premedication in patients for surgery under general anesthesia. Anesthesia, Essays and Researches. 2017;**11**(4):854-858. DOI: 10.4103/aer.AER_106_17

[30] Slatkin NE, Xie F, Messina J, Segal TJ. Fentanyl buccal tablet for relief of breakthrough pain in opioid-tolerant patients with cancer-related chronic pain. The Journal of Supportive Oncology. 2007;**5**(7):327-334

[31] Hashemi M, Zali A, Golmakani E, et al. Efficacy, safety, and tolerability of sublingual fentanyl orally disintegrating tablet in the treatment of breakthrough cancer pain: A randomized, double-blind, placebo-controlled study. Daru. 2021;**29**(1):51-59. DOI: 10.1007/s40199-020-00381-6

[32] Boyer EW. Management of opioid analgesic overdose. The New England Journal of Medicine. 2012;**367**:146-155. DOI: 10.1056/NEJMra1202561

[33] Mann K, Bladström A, Torup L, et al. Extending the treatment options in alcohol dependence: A randomized controlled study of as-needed nalmefene. Biological Psychiatry. 2013;**73**(8):706-713. DOI: 10.1016/j.biopsych.2012.10.020

[34] PAJ J, Gardocki JF. Method for producing analgesia. US Patent 3141823. 21 Jul 1964. Available from: https://patents.google.com/patent/US3141823A/en [Accessed: May 19, 2023]

[35] Braga FC, Ramos TO, Brocksom TJ, de Oliviera KT. Synthesis of fentanyl under continuous photoflow conditions. Organic Letters. 2022;**24**(45):8331-8336. DOI: 10.1021/acs.orglett.2c03338

[36] Zee S-H, Wang W-K. A new process for the synthesis of fentanyl. JCCS. 1980;**27**(4):147-149. DOI: 10.1002/jccs.198000026

[37] Gupta PK, Manral L, Ganesan K, et al. A method for the preparation of fentanyl. European Patent, 2252149A2. 2010. Available from: https://patents.google.com/patent/EP2252149A2/en [Accessed: April 22, 2023]

[38] Cayman. Standardized Naming of Substituted Fentanyls [Internet]. 2018. Available from: https://www.caymanchem.com/news/standardized-naming-of-substituted-fentanyls [Accessed: May 10, 2023]

[39] Valdez CA, Leif RN, Mayer BP. An efficient, optimized synthesis of fentanyl and related analogs. PLoS One. 2014;**9**(9):e108250. DOI: 10.1371/journal.pone.0108250

[40] National Library of Medicine. Fentanyl [Internet]. 2023. Available from: https://pubchem.ncbi.nlm.nih.gov/compound/Fentanyl [Accessed: June 02, 2023]

[41] Wilde M, Pichini S, Pacifici R, et al. Metabolic pathways and potencies of new fentanyl analogs. Frontiers in Pharmacology. 2019;**5**(10):238. DOI: 10.3389/fphar.2019.00238

[42] National Library of Medicine. Alfentanil [Internet]. 2023. Available from: https://pubchem.ncbi.nlm.nih.gov/compound/Alfentanil [Accessed: June 02, 2023]

[43] Lee GM et al. The clinical effective dose of alfentanil for suppressing cough during emergence from desflurane anesthesia. KJA. 2011;**61**(4):292-296. DOI: 10.4097/kjae.2011.61.4.292

[44] Moman RN, Mowery ML, Kelley B. Alfentanil [Internet]. 2022. Available from: https://www.ncbi.nlm.nih.gov/

books/NBK470456/#article-17352.s8 [Accessed: November 13, 2022]

[45] Zhao N, Zeng J, Fan L, Zhang C, Wu Y, Wang X, et al. The effect of alfentanil on emergence delirium following general anesthesia in children: A randomized clinical trial. Paediatric Drugs. 2022;**24**(4):413-421. DOI: 10.1007/s40272-022-00510-5

[46] Drugbank Online. Alfentanil [Internet]. 2023. Available from: https://go.drugbank.com/drugs/DB00802 [Accessed: March 28, 2023]

[47] Westmoreland LC. Pharmacokinetics of remifentanil (GI87084B) and its metabolite (GI90291) in patients undergoing elective inpatient summery. Anesthesiology. 1993;**79**(5):893-903. DOI: 10.1097/00000542-199311000-00005

[48] National Center for Biotechnology Information. PubChem Compound Summary for CID 60815, Remifentanil [Internet]. 2023. Available from: https://pubchem.ncbi.nlm.nih.gov/compound/Remifentanil [Accessed: May 16, 2023]

[49] Servin FS, Billard V. Remifentanil and other opioids. Handbook of Experimental Pharmacology. 2008;**182**:283-311. DOI: 10.1007/978-3-540-74806-9_14

[50] Kurzová A, Málek J, Hess L, et al. Non-traditional administration of remifentanil in an experimental setting. Physiology. 2019;**68**(Suppl. 1):97-103. In Czech Language

[51] National Center for Biotechnology Information. PubChem Compound Summary for CID 41693, Sufentanil [Internet]. 2023. Available from: https://pubchem.ncbi.nlm.nih.gov/compound/Sufentanil [Accessed: May 16, 2023]

[52] Hess L. Nové deriváty fentanylu – carfentanil, lofentanil, sufentanil a alfentanil. Remedia. 1992;**2**(4-5):263-264. ISSN 0862-8947. In Czech Language

[53] Berg A, Habeck J, Strigenz M, et al. Sublingual Sufentanil vs. intravenous fentanyl for the treatment of acute postoperative pain in the ambulatory surgery center: A randomized clinical trial. Anesthesiology Research and Practice. 2022;**2022**:5237877. DOI: 10.1155/2022/5237877

[54] Savoia G, Loreto M, Gravino E. Sufentanil: An overview of its use for acute pain management. Minerva Anesthesiology. 2001;**67**(9):206-216

[55] Zhang C, Huang D, Zeng W, et al. Effect of additional equipotent fentanyl or sufentanil administration on recovery profiles during propofol-remifentanil-based anaesthesia in patients undergoing gynaecologic laparoscopic surgery: A randomized clinical trial. BMC Anesthesiology. 2022;**22**(1):127. DOI: 10.1186/s12871-022-01671-z

[56] National Center for Biotechnology Information. PubChem Compound Summary for CID 62156, Carfentanil. [Internet]. 2023. Available from: https://pubchem.ncbi.nlm.nih.gov/compound/Carfentanil [Accessed: May 16, 2023]

[57] Hess L. Carfentanil – nejsilnější známý opioid. Remedia. 2017;**27**(6):582-586. Available from: https://www.medvik.cz/bmc/link.do?id=bmc18000366 Accessed: May 16, 2023

[58] Leen JLS, Juurlink DN. Carfentanil: A narrative review of its pharmacology and public health concerns. Canadian Journal of Anesthesia. 2019;**66**:414-421. DOI: 10.1007/s12630-019-01294-y

[59] Bhatt N, Nimavat K. Synthesis, characterization and antimicrobial activity of methyl 1-(−2-amine-alkylcarbonyl) piperidine-4-carboxylate. IJPRS. 2013;**2**:11-15

[60] Bilsback P, Rolly G, Tampubolon O. Efficacy of the extradural administration of Lofentanil, buprenorphine or saline in the management of postoperative pain. British Journal of Anaesthesia. 1985;**57**:943-948. DOI: 10.1093/bja/57.10.943

[61] Středa L, Patočka J. Neletální chemické zbraně a Úmluva o zákazu chemických zbraní. Vojenské zdravotnické listy. 2004;**73**(5-6):184-193. In Czech Language

[62] European Monitoring Centre for Drugs and Drug Addiction and Europol. Acryloylfentanyl: EMCDDA–Europol Joint Report on a New Psychoactive Substance: *N*-(1-Phenethylpiperidin-4-yl)-*N*-Phenylacrylamide (Acryloylfentanyl); Lisbon. 2017 [Internet]. 2017. Available from: https://www.emcdda.europa.eu/publications/joint-reports/acryloylfentanyl_en [Accessed: August 23, 2022]

[63] Ujváry I, Jorge R, Christie R, et al. Acryloylfentanyl, a recently emerged new psychoactive substance: A comprehensive review. Forensic Toxicology. 2017;**35**:232-243

[64] UNODC. Fentanyl and its Analogues - 50 Years on [Internet]. 2017. Available from: https://www.unodc.org/documents/scientific/Global_SMART_Update_17_web.pdf [Accessed: August 29, 2021]

[65] The Dangers of Abusing Fentanyl Patches. Drug & Alcohol Rehab Centers [Internet]. 2019. Available from: https://americanaddictioncenters.org/fentanyl-treatment/dangers-of-abuse [Accessed: April 26, 2021]

[66] UNODC. World Drug Report 2022 (United Nations publication, 2022) [Internet]. 2019. Available from: www.unodc.org/unodc/en/data-and-analysis/world-drug-report-2022.html [Accessed: May 26, 2023]

[67] Legislative Assembly of British Columbia. Expanding the Response to the Toxic Drug and Overdose Crisis. [Internet]. 2022. Available from: https://www.leg.bc.ca/content/CommitteeDocuments/42nd-parliament/3rd-session/health/report/SSC-Health-Report_42-3_2022-11-01_Final.pdf [Accessed: June 08, 2023]

[68] Pierce M, van Amsterdam J, Kalkman GA, et al. Is Europe facing an opioid crisis like the United States? An analysis of opioid use and related adverse effects in 19 European countries between 2010 and 2018. European Psychiatry. 2021;**64**(1):e47. DOI: 10.1192/j.eurpsy.2021.2219

[69] Ellis CR, Kruhlak NL, Kim MT, et al. Predicting opioid receptor binding affinity of pharmacologically unclassified designer substances using molecular docking. PLoS One. 2018;**13**(5):e0197734. DOI: 10.1371/journal.pone.0197734

[70] UNODC: World Drug Report 2022 [Internet]. 2022. Available from: https://www.unodc.org/res/wdr2022/MS/WDR22_Booklet_1.pdf [Accessed: April 25, 2023]

[71] US Department of Justice; Drug Enforcement Administration. Schedules of controlled substances: Temporary placement of acetyl fentanyl into schedule I. Federal Register. 2015;**80**:29227-29230

[72] Papsun D, Krywanczyk A, Vose JC, et al. Analysis of MT-45, a novel synthetic opioid, in human whole blood by LC–MS-MS and its identification

in a drug-related death. Journal of Analytical Toxicology. 2016;**40**:313-317. DOI: 10.3390/ijerph16020177

[73] Bäckberg M, Beck O, Jönsson KH, Helander A. Opioid intoxications involving butyrfentanyl, 4-fluorobutyrfentanyl, and fentanyl from the Swedish STRIDA project. Clinical Toxicology. 2015;**53**:609-617. DOI: 10.3109/15563650.2015.1054505

[74] Report of the International Narcotics Control Board [Internet]. 2022. Available from: https://www.unodc.org/documents/treaties/COP11/Other_Relevant_Documentation/E_2022_28-E_CN.7_2022_14_E.pdf [Accessed: January 18, 2023]

[75] Vandeputte MM et al. Phenethyl-4-ANPP: A marginally active byproduct suggesting a switch in illicit fentanyl synthesis routes. Journal of Analytical Toxicology. 2022;**46**(4):350-357. DOI: 10.1093/jat/bkab032

[76] Lovrecic B, Lovrecic M, Gabrovec B, et al. Non-medical use of novel synthetic opioids: A new challenge to public health. IJRPH. 2019;**16**(2):177. DOI: 10.3390/ijerph16020177

[77] Dynex. Drug test. New: Fentanyl test. NPC Bulletin 2013. p. 3 [Internet]. 2013. Available from: https://www.dynex.cz/data/machines/bulletin-npdc-03_2013.pdf [Accessed: August 18, 2017]

[78] Goldman JE, Waye KM, Periera KA, et al. Perspectives on rapid fentanyl test strips as a harm reduction practice among young adults who use drugs: A qualitative study. Harm Reduction Journal. 2019;**16**:3. DOI: 10.1186/s12954-018-0276-0

[79] Jelínková R, Moravcová I, Žuja P. Orientation test for the presence of fentanyl derivatives by thin-layer chromatography. Chemicke Listy. 2023;**117**(3):155-162. DOI: 10.54779/chl20230155

[80] Jelínková R. Extractive spectrophotometry of fentanyl and its derivatives [thesis]. Brno: University of Defence; 2014

[81] Ott CE, Perez-Estebanez M, Hernandez S, et al. Forensic identification of fentanyl and its analogs by electrochemical-surface enhanced Raman spectroscopy (EC-SERS) for the screening of seized drugs of abuse. Frontiers in Analytical Science. 2022;**2**:202. DOI: 10.3389/frans.2022.834820

[82] Travon C, Ott CE, Dalzell KA, et al. Screening of seized drugs utilizing portable Raman spectroscopy and direct analysis in real time-mass spectrometry (DART-MS). Forensic Chemistry. 2021;**25**:1000352. DOI: 10.1016/j.forc.2021.100352

[83] Choińska MK, Šestáková I, Hrdlička V, et al. Electroanalysis of fentanyl and its new analogs: A review. Biosensors (Basel). 2022;**12**(1):26. DOI: 10.3390/bios12010026

[84] UNODC – United Nations Office on Drugs and Crime. Recommended Methods for the Identification and Analysis Od Fentanyl and its Analogues in Biological Specimens. The United Nations in Vienna; 2017

[85] Maher S, Elliot SP, George S. The analytical challenges of cyklopropylfentanyl and crotonylfentanyl: An approach for toxicological analysis. Drug Testing and Analysis. 2018;**10**(9):1493-1487. DOI: 10.1002/dta.2417

[86] Marchei E, Pacifici R, Mannocchi G, et al. New synthetic opioids in biological

and non-biological matrices: A review of current analytical methods. TrAC Trends in Analytical Chemistry. 2018;**102**:1-15. DOI: 10.1016/j.trac.2018.01.007

[87] Roda G, Faggiani F, Bolchi C, et al. Ten years of fentanyl-like drugs: A technical-analytical review. Analytical Sciences. 2019;**35**:479-491. DOI: 10.2116/analsci.18R004

[88] Strayer EK et al. LC-MS/MS-based method for the multiplex detection of 24 fentanyl analogues and metabolites in whole blood at sub ng.mL^{-1} concentrations. ACS. Omega. 2018;**3**(1):514-523. DOI: 10.1021/acsomega.7b01536

[89] Riches RJ et al. Analysis of clothing and urine from Moscow theatre siege casualties reveals Carfentanil and remifentanil use. Journal of Analytical Toxicology. 2012;**36**(9):647-656. DOI: 10.1093/jat/bks078

[90] Halámek E, Kobliha Z. Potential chemical warfare agents. Chemicke Listy. 2011;**105**(5):323-333

[91] Kobliha Z, Středa L. Neletální chemické zbraně – zbraně pro 21. století? Brno; 2015 ISBN: 978-80-263-0975-8

[92] Pearson A. Incapacitating biochemical wapons. Nonprolferation Review. 2006;**13**(2):151-188. DOI: 10.1080/10736700601012029

[93] Pitschmann V, Hon Z. Drugs as chemical weapons: Past and perspectives. Toxics. 2023;**11**(1):52. DOI: 10.3390/toxics11010052

Chapter 5

Opioids in Cancer Therapy: Benefits, Risks, and Critical Challenges

Parisa Saberi-Hasanabadi, Milad Esmaeilzadeh Farmad, Amin Ataie and Ramin Ataee

Abstract

Pain management in cancer patients is one of the main components of palliative treatment. The requirement for rational use of opioids is careful selection of patients, correct prescription of these compounds, compliance with drug dosage, regular sequence of use, compliance with side effects, and drug interactions. Most cancer patients with moderate to severe pain will respond to treatment with opioid analgesics. Limited comprehensive studies have been conducted so far on the use of opioids in cancer pain management. In this chapter, databases for the search included PubMed, MedLine, and Embase databases along with reviews and cross-references. We examine the continuous use of opioids and the related consequences and challenges in the management of patients with cancer pain. In addition, the discussion includes the therapeutic use of opioids, the effectiveness of treatment with this group of compounds, the assessment of the risk of continuous opioid use, and the guidance for administration of opioids in patients with cancer. In general, the effects of opioid use in different age groups with on cancer progression, metastases, and recurrence can be an interesting indication that is worth future research in case of loss of analgesic response in time.

Keywords: opioid therapy, cancer, pain management, outcomes, pharmacology aspects

1. Introduction

Most cancer patients experience pain. Many of them require opioids to relieve their pain during the course of treatment, and these compounds remain the most effective form of pain relief [1]. According to the estimates of the International Association for the Study of Pain, the prevalence of pain in all types of cancer ranges from 20 to 89% [2]. The intensity of pain varies depending on cancer subtype, treatments received, pain metric, and time since completion of oncological therapy [3]. For example, persistent pain after surgical treatment has been found to be very common in women with breast cancer. The prevalence and increasing trend of pain is higher among young patients undergoing radiotherapy and dissection of axillary lymph nodes. About 20 to 50% of women are affected by persistent neuropathic pain after surgical treatment. Prescription of opioid drugs is the treatment of choice to relieve chronic pain caused by advanced cases of cancer [4]. Various approaches for pain management and treatment are given in (**Table 1**). The requirement for the rational use of these drugs is careful selection of patients, correct prescription of opioid drugs, compliance with drug dosage, regular sequence of use, compliance with side effects, and drug interactions. Prescription and consumption of opioids to cancer patients are inadequate and do not have a regular pattern [7]. The effect of opioids on cancer progression, metastases, and recurrence is increasingly being questioned. In order to optimize the pain control of cancer patients, more educational and promotional measures are needed. For this purpose, the step-by-step treatment proposed by the World Health Organization is a good guide as the most appropriate standard treatment guideline for the pain of cancer patients (**Figure 1**). This treatment process starts with the administration of non-opioid drugs, such as paracetamol and ibuprofen. If sufficient analgesia is not achieved, weak opioids, such as codeine and tramadol, should be used. If the pain is still not properly controlled, stronger opioids, such as morphine and oxycodone, can be prescribed [9].

Approaches	Treatment
Modification of underlying pathology	Surgery, chemotherapy, radiotherapy, and hormone therapy.
Pharmacotherapy	Nonsteroidal anti-inflammatory drugs, anticonvulsants, opioids, antidepressants, and corticosteroids.
Interventional techniques	Local anesthetics and neurolytic agents
Non-opioids	Paracetamol, acetyl salicylic acid, indomethacin, ibuprofen, diclofenac, and naproxen.
Weak opioids for mild to moderate pain	Codeine, tramadol, and dihydrocodeine
Strong opioids for moderate to severe pain	Morphine, methadone, and oxycodone

Table 1.
Different approaches to cancer pain management [5, 6].

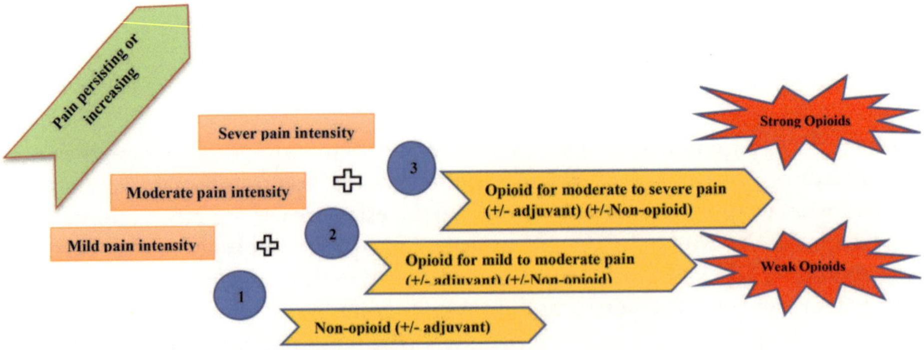

Figure 1.
WHO's analgesic ladder for relief of cancer pain [8].

The purpose of this review was to examine the reasons and current status of prescribing and consuming opioids in patients with advanced cancer and to provide solutions to rationalize this process.

2. Methods

In this chapter, we will discuss the prevalence of chronic cancer pain, the therapeutic use of opioids, the effectiveness of treatment with this class of therapeutic compounds, guidance for the responsible and consistent administration of opioids for patients with chronic cancer, associated outcomes, and the challenges of managing patients with chronic cancer pain. The comprehensive literature search was conducted for the period 2004 through June 2023. Databases for this purpose included PubMed, EMBASE, Cochrane reviews, and clinicaltrails.gov along with reviews and cross-references. Keywords in this search focused on opioid therapy in the management of cancer-related pain. All studies were independently screened and reviewed by the authors based on their titles and abstracts. The full text of articles potentially suitable for review was assessed.

3. Opioids

3.1 Pharmacology aspects

As mentioned, opioid therapy is often used to control pain in most cancer patients during their disease course. Opioids are the cornerstone of pain management in cancer treatment, and their use has been increasing in recent years. Cancer pain is usually effectively treated by administering opioids at regular intervals and providing effective doses to manage pain failure [9]. No specific opioid will be prescribed for all patients. It is possible to optimize the effect of an opioid for any manifestation of the disease [10, 11]. Specialists are not able to predict the exact treatment response of patients. After the initial opioid administration, its clinical effectiveness may decrease gradually over time or even suddenly, resulting in the need to increase the dose. In some cases, increasing the dose does not cause pain relief and may even cause side effects [12, 13].

The proper administration of opioids, considering their wide range, requires a deep understanding of the pharmacology and pharmacokinetics of these different analgesics. Opioids cause analgesia by acting on receptors located in the membrane of nerve cells. Their main effect in the nervous system is the presynaptic effect in inhibiting the release of neurotransmitters [6]. There are three types of opioid receptors, including m, d, and k (mu, delta, and kappa) [7]. Understanding the molecular structure of opiate receptors will lead to the provision of more accurate approaches in the study of opioid pharmacology (**Figure 2**). Opioid receptors are found throughout the body, mainly in the brain, spinal cord, and intestinal tract. These receptors consist of complex structures of seven amino acid chains, each of which is placed on the membrane and forms a channel that can allow calcium ions to pass inside or outside the neuron [9]. Pharmacological studies have shown that the interaction of the natural opioid-like peptide, b-endorphin, is preferentially with m-receptors, enkephalins with d-receptors, and dynorphin with k-receptors (**Table 2**).

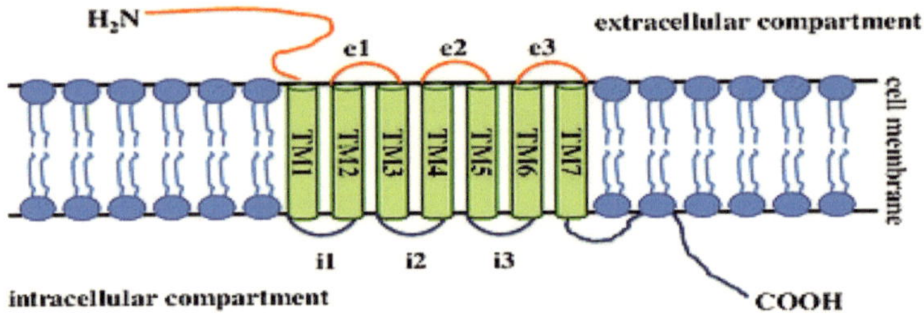

Figure 2.
Opioid receptor structure [14].

The affinity of morphine is more concentrated at m-receptors compared to other opioid receptors. The opioid antagonist naloxone results in the inhibition of all opioid receptors, but its greatest affinity is focused on m-receptors. By connecting an opioid substance to each of these three types of receptors, they cause analgesia. Activation of k- receptors does not cause physical dependence as much as activation of m-receptors [7, 19]. Pure opioid agonists, such as morphine, hydromorphone, and

No	Design	Regular opioids	Severe adverse effects	Follow-up	Ref.
1	A prospective survey of inpatients and outpatients on regularly dosed morphine	Morphine	Dry mouth, sedation, and constipation were frequent, nausea, Myoclonus.	4 weeks	[15]
2	An observational study	Tapentadol and oxycodone/ naloxone	Higher rates of erythema and vomiting, especially in females.	–	[16]
3	A prospective, real-world, and multinational study	Naloxegol	Treatment-related adverse events were mainly gastrointestinal events, the most frequently reported being abdominal pain and diarrhea.	4 weeks	[17]
4	A prospective single-center observational study	Nalbuphine and Morphine	Nalbuphine therapy was accompanied by a statistically significantly lower incidence of side effects such as skin pruritus, constipation, and micturition disorders compared to morphine ($p < 0.05$).	Two years between March 2019 and March 2020.	[18]

Table 2.
Summary of published opioids-based side effects studies on cancer pain.

fentanyl, stimulate μ-receptors and are considered to be the strongest pain relievers. Opioids with different potency may react with N-methyl-D-aspartate (NMDA) receptors and activate the descending pain pathways of serotonin and noradrenaline from the brainstem. Stimulation of these NMDA receptors may lead to neuropathic pain and tolerance [20–22].

3.2 Common opioid analgesics in cancer pain relief

This work summarizes the current knowledge regarding the impact of common opioids in cancer pain progression with an emphasis on clinical outcomes (**Figure 3**).

3.2.1 Morphine

Morphine is still used as one of the most common pain relievers and cancer pain relievers. Morphine affects the u- and κ-receptors, but its analgesic effect is mainly carried out by the u-receptors [7, 9]. In a randomized, multicenter, and open-label trial at a Japanese hospital's palliative care service, Matsuoka et al., evaluated the potential of the opioid choice in cancer pain management using a catechol-O-methyltransferase (COMT) genotype biomarker. They demonstrated that the proportion of patients requiring high-dose opioids was significantly higher in the morphine group when compared with the oxycodone group in those with the COMT-rs4680 GG genotype [23]. Wasan et al., stated that hydromorphone was present in 66% of morphine users without aberrant drug behavior. This proves that morphine is metabolized to codeine and hydromorphone in small amounts. This process usually occurs with doses higher than 100 mg per day [24].

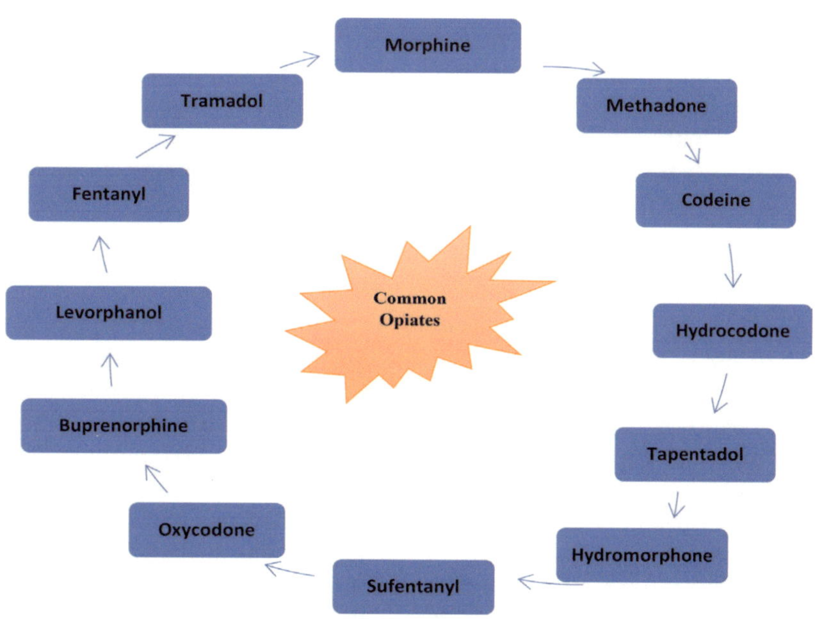

Figure 3.
Common opioid compounds during clinical use [7, 9].

3.2.2 Codeine

Codeine is known as a prodrug and a weak opioid. Generally, this opioid is prescribed after surgery and is used along with specific medications to manage acute and chronic pain. Its administration is not recommended in the presence of renal failure. Codeine administration in children had low clinical effectiveness and has not shown a significant response with increasing the dosage [9]. Ou et al., stated that short-term use of tramadol compared with codeine did not lead to an increased risk of cardiac events among patients with non-cancer pain [25]. Limited literature were found on the effect of codeine on the process of pain management in cancer patients. In this line, Straube et al., investigated the efficacy and safety of codeine used alone or in combination with paracetamol for relieving cancer pain. Overall, codeine or codeine plus paracetamol was numerically superior to placebo groups and equivalent to active comparators [26].

3.2.3 Hydrocodone

Like codeine, it has been proposed that hydrocodone is a prodrug used in patients with advanced cancer. Today, hydrocodone is available as an extended-release with side effects similar to other opioids. This opioid is a suitable option for children who have a poorly metabolized phenotype [27].

3.2.4 Hydromorphone

The structure of hydromorphone is similar to morphine, and it is available in both oral and injectable forms [27]. Its high potency and solubility may be useful for patients who require high doses of opioids injected subcutaneously [9]. In a review study, Li et al., stated that hydromorphone to work as well as morphine, oxycodone, and fentanyl and appears to be an alternative opioid analgesic, which may help relieve pain symptoms for people with advanced cancer. This review includes a total of eight studies, which compared hydromorphone with oxycodone, morphine, and fentanyl. They found no clear evidence of a difference in nausea, vomiting, and dizziness in persons treated with hydromorphone compared with those treated with morphine [28]. The evidence is very uncertain and no studies reporting quality of life. Also, these studies did not include children.

3.2.5 Fentanyl

Fentanyl is approximately 80 times more potent than morphine, and as a highly lipophilic opioid is used for relieving cancer pain in transdermal and transmucosal immediate-release formulations [7]. Fentanyl undergoes extensive metabolism in the liver and binds strongly to plasma proteins. It is one of the most commonly used analgesics among pediatric patients. Fentanyl can be administered by continuous intravenous or subcutaneous infusion [9]. Thantiprechapong et al., evaluated the efficacy of reconstituted intravenous rapid-acting fentanyl formulations to sublingual solution versus oral morphine for breakthrough pain among patients with chronic gynecologic cancer pain. The primary outcome was the reduction in early breakthrough pain with administration of intravenous fentanyl to sublingual solution. Intravenous fentanyl to sublingual solution may be considered for breakthrough pain when rapid-acting fentanyl formulations are unavailable [29].

3.2.6 Sufentanyl

Sufentanyl is injected into cancer patients as an alternative to fentanyl under certain conditions. A lower dose of sufentanyl is effective for pain control among patients, especially those with renal failure [27]. Tan et al., investigated the postoperative effects of sufentanil preemptive analgesia combined with psychological support therapy on breast cancer patients undergoing radical surgery. Overall, they concluded that prophylactic analgesia with sufentanil administration along with psychological support is an effective method of pain relief for breast cancer patients undergoing radical surgery. This technique deserves to be promoted in the clinic [30].

3.2.7 Methadone

Methadone as a synthetic opioid with highly variable pharmacokinetics is commonly used as a second-line option in the presence of neuropathic pain in cancer. Its average half-life ranges from less than 15 hours to more than 130 hours. The analgesic effect of methadone is more stable than that of morphine. Due to the limited researches in the field of methadone use, the effective dose of this opiate is still a challenging issue and needs to be started, adjusted and carefully monitored during the treatment of cancer patients [31]. In this line, Furst reviewed the current knowledge of low-dose methadone treatment in palliative cancer care. He stated that methadone use requires an experienced physician and solid follow-up. Continuous administration of low-dose methadone has been shown to be effective and safe in reducing pain in dying patients without increasing confusion, regardless of age [32]. Although the available data are not sufficient to draw a final conclusion, observational and controlled studies in the administration of other strong opioids have shown that methadone is a valuable drug even as the first choice in steps two and three of the analgesic ladder.

3.2.8 Levorphanol

Similar to methadone and morphine, levorphanol is an effective treatment for chronic neuropathic pain. Levorphanol has a shorter plasma half-life with a more prolonged duration of action compared to methadone and may have a substantially lower medication accumulation risk [9, 27]. There are no well-known and extensive studies on the effectiveness of levorphanol in cancer patients, and current evidence is not insufficient to support its use in many pain situations. Reddy et al., determined the proportion of successful opioid rotation from morphine equivalent daily dose to levorphanol in cancer patients with successful opioid rotation. The obtained preliminary data showed that cancer patients could be successfully rotated to levorphanol using an opioid rotation ratio of 8.5. Levorphanol administration was associated with improvement of pain and disease symptoms control and was well-tolerated [33].

3.2.9 Buprenorphine

Buprenorphine has been used for many years to relieve acute pain and more recently to treat opioid addiction and relieve chronic pain. It has a high affinity for the u-receptor and is used for managing cancer pain with conversion to an active metabolite called norbuprenorphine, which is a weaker but full-opioid agonist [9, 27]. Shen et al., monitored the effects of transdermal buprenorphine on quality of life and some effective symptoms in cancer patients with pain in Asian populations. The preliminary evidence from the administration of transdermal buprenorphine showed an improvement in the quality of life and a reduction in the severity of symptoms and pain in Asian patients with cancer [34].

3.2.10 Oxycodone

Oxycodone is an oral and semisynthetic opioid used to relieve cancer-related pain. Administration of oxycodone was more effective in reducing pain intensity than other strong opioids and resulted in fewer side effects, indicating a better effect of this drug in pain relief in cancer patients [20]. King et al., reviewed the quality of evidence for the use of oxycodone in the relief of cancer pain in adults. There was no evidence of a significant difference in analgesia or side effects between oxycodone and either morphine or hydromorphone. Therefore, oxycodone can be used as a suitable alternative to morphine or hydromorphone in cancer-related pain [35]. In this line, Weme et al., evaluated the potential drug-drug interaction of enzalutamide and oxycodone in men with prostate cancer. Co-administration of enzalutamide showed a significant decrease in exposure to oxycodone and its active metabolite oxymorphone, which should be considered when prescribing enzalutamide with oxycodone [36].

3.2.11 Tramadol

Tramadol is recommended for cancer patients with moderate to severe pain when other opioids are ineffective. Tramadol contains two enantiomers and a synthetic analog of codeine and morphine, both of which increase analgesic properties through different mechanisms [37]. Tuan et al., evaluated the role of tramadol/dexketoprofen fixed-dose combination in management of patients with moderate-to-severe acute cancer pain. The pharmacological synergism between tramadol and dexketoprofen along with the environmental effect compared to the use of each of these medicinal compounds alone will lead to an increase in analgesic activity in lower doses and with better tolerance [37].

3.2.12 Tapentadol

Tapentadol is structurally similar to tramadol and is used to relieve severe chronic pain in cancer patients [9]. Boland et al., suggested that tapentadol as an effective pain reliever can be used as an alternative to morphine and oxycodone, especially during opioid poisoning [38]. In a prospective, multicenter, open-label study, Jung et al., monitored the clinical efficacy of tapentadol on pain control and the quality of life of patients with moderate to severe chronic cancer pain in clinical practice in Korea. They stated that tapentadol extended-release was effective for treating patients with moderate to severe cancer pain and neuropathic pain, and therefore it significantly improved the patients' quality of life [39].

3.3 Opioid routes of administration

Opioids should be administered in the least invasive and safest way possible to achieve satisfactory analgesia. Oral administration is preferred over other routes because of its convenience, relative safety, and cheapness. An accepted alternative for long-term treatment is the use of the transdermal route [7, 9]. Some of the most important routes of opioid administration are shown in (**Figure 4**).

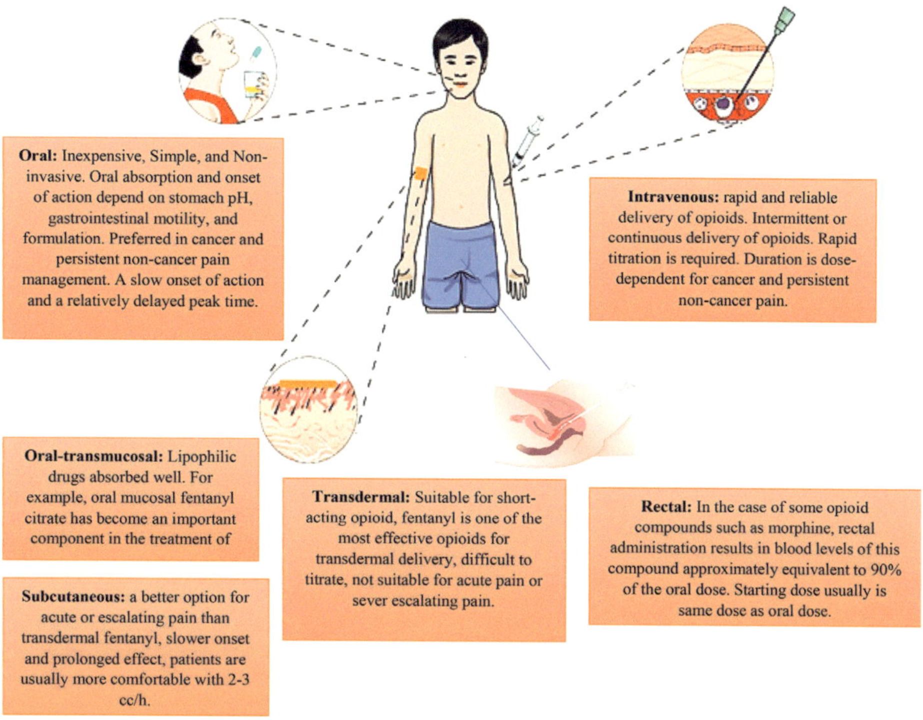

Figure 4.
Opioid routes of administration [7, 9, 27].

3.4 Mechanism of action in pain relief

Major recent advances in understanding the mechanism of action of opioids include the cloning and identification of opioid receptors (opioid receptors), understanding the cellular function of opioids, and identifying the sites of opioid action in the brain. With the activation of the receptor, the protein released inside the cell leads to the activation of Na/K channels and affecting intracellular enzymes or nuclear gene transcription [9]. Opioid receptors can be presynaptic or postsynaptic. Presynaptic opioid receptors inhibit the release of neurotransmitters acetylcholine, norepinephrine, and serotonin [7].

3.5 Factors influencing outcomes

Studies have shown that factors, such as age, gender, pain syndrome, and the use of auxiliary drugs, did not affect the need for opioids or their replacement. This is while underlying diseases such as kidney failure along with the use of certain drugs caused a change in opioids and their effective dose in pain relief [19]. The results in this field are somewhat contradictory.

3.6 Risks and side effects

As with any potential therapy, opioids carry risks and adverse effects. The use of opioids causes various side effects at the same time as the administration of chemotherapy drugs, most of which include nausea and vomiting, constipation, and depression [7, 27]. In some circumstances, some patients avoid opioids because of these side effects, which may act as an important barrier to complete pain relief (**Table 2**).

4. Conclusions and future perspective

Pain relief guidelines have been developed to care for patients after surgery and improve their quality of life. Cancer patients usually undergo chemotherapy, which can be painful and uncomfortable. Therefore, patients need to use opioids. It is very important to have correct information about the patient's pharmacogenomics during pain management and medical care. In order to optimize research in this field, prospective studies should include experimental designs, randomized and controlled clinical trials on cancer pain patients receiving opioids and control patients. Others include pre- and posttreatment assessments, adequate sample sizes, and neuropsychological testing that can be related to opioid use. Examination of patient quality of life, mechanisms by which different opioids may affect cognition, opioid switching/rotation, short-acting opioids on demand, individual differences/characteristics/genetics, emotional factors, and other symptoms should not be overlooked. Switching from one opioid to another may be problematic, especially when using high doses. Unpredictable conversion rates depend on many individual and clinical variables. Some opiates, such as methadone, are suitable compounds due to their much lower cost, which is a great advantage in developing countries. Of course, in the use of these compounds, attention should be paid to their pharmacokinetics as an increase in the risk of accumulation and delayed toxicity, apart from the potential for this compound to interact with other drugs. The limitations of the studies used and sometimes their quality are obvious limitations in writing this chapter. In addition, there is limited information on dose titration methods for each opioid. The concern of using these compounds in the pediatric population and people with underlying diseases can be an interesting indication that is worth future research. Further studies with appropriate design should provide information on the long-term use of opioids with the previously mentioned details.

Conflict of interest

The authors declared no conflict of interest.

DOI: http://dx.doi.org/10.5772/intechopen.112852

Author details

Parisa Saberi-Hasanabadi[1], Milad Esmaeilzadeh Farmad[2], Amin Ataie[3] and Ramin Ataee[4,5,6]*

1 Department of Toxicology and Pharmacology, Faculty of Pharmacy, Mazandaran University of Medical Sciences, Sari, Iran

2 Orthopedic Surgeon Center at the 9th Dey of Torbat Heydariyeh Hospital, Mashhad University of Medical Sciences, Iran

3 Cellular and Molecular Research Center, Babol University of Medical Sciences, Babol, Iran

4 Pharmaceutical Science Research Center, Hemoglobinopathy Institute, Mazandaran University of Medical Sciences, Sari, Iran

5 Medicinal Plants Research Center, Mazandaran University of Medical Sciences, Sari, Iran

6 Thalassemia Research Center, Hemoglobinopathy Institute, Mazandaran University of Medical Sciences, Sari, Iran

*Address all correspondence to: raminataee1349@gmail.com

IntechOpen

© 2024 The Author(s). Licensee IntechOpen. This chapter is distributed under the terms of the Creative Commons Attribution License (http://creativecommons.org/licenses/by/3.0), which permits unrestricted use, distribution, and reproduction in any medium, provided the original work is properly cited.

References

[1] Sun M, Chang CL, Lu CY, Zhang J, Wu SY. Effect of opioids on cancer survival in patients with chronic pain: A propensity score-matched population-based cohort study. British Journal of Anaesthesia. 2022;**128**(4):708-717

[2] Van den Beuken-van Everdingen MHJ, De Rijke JM, Kessels AG, Schouten HC, Van Kleef M, Patijn J. Prevalence of pain in patients with cancer: A systematic review of the past 40 years. Annals of Oncology. 2007;**18**(9):1437-1449

[3] Preux C, Bertin M, Tarot A, Authier N, Pinol N, Brugnon D, et al. Prevalence of opioid use disorder among patients with cancer-related pain: A systematic review. Journal of Clinical Medicine. 2022;**11**(6):1594

[4] Satija A, Ahmed SM, Gupta R, Ahmed A, Rana SPS, Singh SP, et al. Breast cancer pain management-A review of current & novel therapies. The Indian Journal of Medical Research. 2014;**139**(2):216

[5] World Health Organization. National Cancer Control Programmes: Policies and Managerial Guidelines. World Health Organization; 2002

[6] Dalal S, Bruera E. Access to opioid analgesics and pain relief for patients with cancer. Nature Reviews Clinical Oncology. 2013;**10**(2):108-116

[7] Trescot AM. Opioid pharmacology and pharmacokinetics. Controlled Substance Management in Chronic Pain: A Balanced Approach. 2016:45-62

[8] Ferreira ASL, Kimura M, Jacobsen Teixeira M. The WHO analgesic ladder for cancer pain control, twenty years of use. How much pain relief does one get from using it? Supportive Care in Cancer. 2006;**14**:1086-1093

[9] Subramaniam V, Salem Yehya AH, Oon CE. Molecular basis of cancer pain management: An updated review. Medicina. 2019;**55**(9):584

[10] Colson J, Koyyalagunta D, Falco F, Manchikanti L. A systematic review of observational studies on the effectiveness of opioid therapy for cancer pain. Pain Physician. 2011;**14**(2):E85

[11] Manchikanti L, Manchikanti KN, Kaye AD, Kaye AM, Hirsch JA. Challenges and concerns of persistent opioid use in cancer patients. Expert Review of Anticancer Therapy. 2018;**18**(7):705-718

[12] Friesen C, Bacher S, Hormann I, Roscher M, Miltner E. Cytotoxic effects of opioids on cancer cell lines. International Journal of Clinical Pharmacology and Therapeutics. 2011;**49**(1):60

[13] Bennett M, Paice JA, Wallace M. Pain and opioids in cancer care: Benefits, risks, and alternatives. American Society of Clinical Oncology Educational Book. 2017;**37**:705-713

[14] Sobczak M, Sałaga M, Storr MA, Fichna J. Physiology, signaling, and pharmacology of opioid receptors and their ligands in the gastrointestinal tract: Current concepts and future perspectives. Journal of Gastroenterology. 2014;**49**:24-45

[15] Glare P, Walsh D, Sheehan D. The adverse effects of morphine: A prospective survey of common symptoms during repeated dosing for

chronic cancer pain. American Journal of Hospice and Palliative Medicine®. 2006;**23**(3):229-235

[16] Shi C, Liu J, Hu J, Chen X, Xie J, Luo J, et al. Genetic and clinical factors associated with opioid response in Chinese Han patients with cancer pain: An exploratory cross-sectional study. Pain and therapy. 2022;**11**(1):269-288

[17] Davies A, Cinieri S, Dupoiron D, España Fernandez S, Leclerc J, Montesarchio V, et al. A prospective, real-world, multinational study of Naloxegol for patients with cancer pain diagnosed with opioid-induced constipation—The NACASY study. Cancers. 2022;**14**(5):1128

[18] Kubica-Cielińska A, Czapla M, Juárez-Vela R, Tejada-Garrido CI, Zielińska M. Comparison of side effects of nalbuphine and morphine in the treatment of pain in children with cancer: A prospective study. Cancers. 2022;**14**(15):3617

[19] Mercadante S, Bruera E. Opioid switching in cancer pain: From the beginning to nowadays. Critical Reviews in Oncology/Hematology. 2016;**99**:241-248

[20] Kaplan R, Parris WC, Citron ML, Zhukovsky D, Reder RF, Buckley BJ, et al. Comparison of controlled-release and immediate-release oxycodone tablets in patients with cancer pain. Journal of Clinical Oncology. 1998;**16**(10):3230-3237

[21] Constance JE, Campbell SC, Somani AA, Yellepeddi V, Owens KH, Sherwin CM. Pharmacokinetics, pharmacodynamics and pharmacogenetics associated with nonsteroidal anti-inflammatory drugs and opioids in pediatric cancer patients. Expert Opinion on Drug Metabolism & Toxicology. 2017;**13**(7):715-724

[22] Meldrum ML. A capsule history of pain management. JAMA. 2003;**290**(18):2470-2475

[23] Matsuoka H, Tsurutani J, Chiba Y, Fujita Y, Sakai K, Yoshida T, et al. Morphine versus oxycodone for cancer pain using a catechol-O-methyltransferase genotype biomarker: A multicenter, randomized, open-label, phase III clinical trial (RELIEF Study). The Oncologist. 2023;**28**(3):278-e166

[24] Wasan AD, Michna E, Janfaza D, Greenfield S, Teter CJ, Jamison RN. Interpreting urine drug tests: Prevalence of morphine metabolism to hydromorphone in chronic pain patients treated with morphine. Pain Medicine. 2008;**9**(7):918-923

[25] Ou LB, Azoulay L, Reynier P, Platt RW, Yoon S, Grad R, et al. Tramadol versus codeine and the short-term risk of cardiovascular events in patients with non-cancer pain: A population-based cohort study. British Journal of Clinical Pharmacology. 2022;**88**(4):1824-1834

[26] Straube C, Derry S, Jackson KC, Wiffen PJ, Bell RF, Strassels S, et al. Codeine, alone and with paracetamol (acetaminophen), for cancer pain. Cochrane Database of Systematic Reviews. 2014;(9)

[27] Prommer EE. Pharmacological management of cancer-related pain. Cancer Control. 2015;**22**(4):412-425

[28] Li Y, Ma J, Lu G, Dou Z, Knaggs R, Xia J, et al. Hydromorphone for cancer pain. Cochrane Database of Systematic Reviews. 2021;**8**

[29] Thantiprechapong T, Tilagul T, Vasikasin V. Efficacy of reconstituted intravenous fentanyl to sublingual solution versus oral morphine syrup for breakthrough pain among patients

with chronic gynecologic cancer pain: A randomized, double-blind, placebo-controlled trial. Journal of Obstetrics and Gynaecology Research. 2023;**2023**

[30] Tan H, Wang C, Jiang Y, Shi Q, Liang W, Li D. Postoperative effect of sufentanil preemptive analgesia combined with psychological intervention on breast cancer patients. BMC Anesthesiology. 2023;**23**(1):170

[31] Mercadante S, Bruera E. Methadone as a first-line opioid in cancer pain management: A systematic review. Journal of Pain and Symptom Management. 2018;**55**(3):998-1003

[32] Fürst P. The use of low-dose methadone as add-on to ongoing opioid treatment in palliative cancer care—An underrated treatment? Life. 2022;**12**(5):679

[33] Reddy A, Haider A, Arthur J, Hui D, Dalal S, Dev R, et al. Levorphanol as a second line opioid in cancer patients presenting to an outpatient supportive care center: An open-label study. Journal of Pain and Symptom Management. 2023;**65**(6):683-690

[34] Shen WC, Hou MM, Huang TL, Wang CH, Huang YM, Chen JS, et al. Transdermal buprenorphine improves overall quality of life and symptom severity in cancer patients with pain. Journal of Clinical Nursing. 2023;**32**(3-4):539-547

[35] King SJ, Reid C, Forbes K, Hanks G. A systematic review of oxycodone in the management of cancer pain. Palliative Medicine. 2011;**25**(5):454-470

[36] Weme DO, Hulskotte LMG, Vervenne WL, Imholz ALT, Cremers RGHM, et al. Enzalutamide reduces oxycodone exposure in men with prostate cancer. Clinical Pharmacokinetics. 2023;**2023**:1-8

[37] Tuan J, Wang EH, De Leon JRC, Mendoza MJ, Varrassi G, De Leon JR. Management of acute cancer pain in Asia: An expert opinion on the role of tramadol/Dexketoprofen fixed-dose combination. Cureus. 2023;**15**(3)

[38] Boland JW. Tapentadol for the management of cancer pain in adults: An update. Current Opinion in Supportive and Palliative Care. 2023;**17**(2):90-97

[39] Jung JY, Chon HJ, Choi YJ, Yeon SE, Choi SY, Lee KH. A prospective, multicenter, open-label study of the clinical efficacy of tapentadol extended-release in the treatment of cancer-related pain and improvement in the quality of life of opioid-naïve or opioid-resistant patients. Supportive Care in Cancer. 2022;**30**(7):6103-6112

Chapter 6

Ten Quality Improvement Initiatives to Standardize Healthcare Processes

Mohammed M. Albaadani, Adel Omar Bataweel, Alaa Mahmoud Ismail, Jameelah Mohammed Yaqoob, Ebrahim Sarwi Asiri, Hesham Ahmed Eid, Khaled M. Kasasbeh, Mohamed Fathy Shaban, Nasr Ali Mohammed, Samir Mohammed Bawazir, Siham Mohammed Saleh and Yasser Sami Amer

Abstract

Quality improvement is a continuous journey to standardize healthcare processes and structure to reduce variation, achieve predictable results, and improve outcomes for patients, healthcare systems, and organizations. Improving quality is about making health care safe, effective, patient-centered, timely, efficient, and equitable. It's about giving the people closest to problems affecting care quality the time, permission, skills, and resources they need to solve them. Patient safety it's a fundamental principle of excellent patient care. On the other hand, patient safety it's a fundamental principle of excellent patient care. Patient safety also is one of the key components of the Institute of Medicine's (IOM) six domains of healthcare quality (Safe, Timely, Effective, Efficient, Equitable, and Patient-centered) that is used as a metric to evaluate how safe is the practice. This work aims to highlight the main quality improvement initiatives, and tools used to standardize healthcare processes and improve patient safety.

Keywords: patient safety, variation, performance improvement, quality initiatives, standardization, patient outcomes, continuous quality improvement

1. Introduction

The healthcare system is designed to produce health, but it may do the opposite and cause harm. There are many factors influencing the likelihood of error. These factors include medical device design, the volume of tasks, the unity and clarity of guidelines and policies, the behavior of others focusing on strategies that maximize the frequency of things going right, the dependency of healthcare providers on one another, the diversity of patients, clinicians and other staff, the vulnerability of patients, variations in the physical layout of clinical environments, variability or lack of regulations, implementation of new technology, the diversity of care pathways and organizations involved [1, 2]. These factors not only increase the vulnerability of patient harm but also make the healthcare system very complex and chaotic. Therefore, there is an urgent need for feasible solutions to cope with these challenges and standardize healthcare processes, making the health system safe, effective, and more efficient. Quality improvement initiatives play a key role in enhancing the quality of processes in hospitals and improving patient safety outcomes. By implementing evidence-based practices and clinical guidelines, healthcare organizations can ensure that patients receive appropriate and effective therapies that are tailored to their individual needs [3]. Quality improvement is defined as a systematic approach that is guided by data to improve health services and the quality of care and outcomes for patients based on iterative change, continuous testing and measurement, and empowerment of frontline teams [4]. It is also defined as the monitoring, assessing, and enhancement of quality healthcare standards as well as the implementation of a series of rigorous, systematic, organization-wide processes that result in measurable improvement in healthcare services [5]. On the other hand, continuous quality improvement (CQI) is defined as a progressive incremental improvement of processes, safety, and patient care [6]. The concept of CQI originated in Japan after World War II and was used extensively in the industrial and manufacturing sectors and has been utilized in the health sector [7, 8]. Over several years, continuous quality improvement has evolved rapidly, and many methodologies have been developed to guide organizations toward streamlining their processes, reducing waste, and improving efficiency. There are many quality improvement tools and approaches which include clinical audit; Plan, Do, Study, Act; model for improvement; LEAN/Six Sigma; performance benchmarking, process mapping, and statistical process control [9].

2. Methodology

For this chapter, we conducted thorough research using a comprehensive literature search approach. We explored internet-based bibliographic databases such as Google™ Scholar and PubMed, as well as direct websites of reputable peer-reviewed journals, books, training courses, programs, and reference websites Joint Commission International (JCI), International Society for Quality in Healthcare (ISQua), and Institute of Healthcare Improvement (IHI) related to healthcare quality, safety, and improvement research. Our specific search terms included but were not limited to "patient safety," "healthcare quality," "health care quality," "evidence-based healthcare," "quality improvement," "improvement research," "implementation research," "quality of health care," "practice guidelines," "clinical audit," "accreditation," "care bundles," "patient care bundle" "continuous quality management," "management, total quality," and "education." Initially, we found 230 results and refined our reference list to approximately 150 highly relevant to our chapter's focus. Further screening excluded resources not aligned with the scope, resulting in a final list of 65 citations included in this chapter.

3. What is variation?

Since this chapter seeks to provide some tools to reduce variation that could affect the outcome of provided care services, it is very important to shed light on this concept. Variation means deviation from the norm. In clinical practice, variation means differences in healthcare processes or outcomes, compared to peers or a gold standard such as an evidence-based guideline recommendation [10]. Variations in healthcare are wide-ranging and can include an array of different treatment options, diagnostic procedures, and medication dosages. Variation is not necessarily bad, and it can be good as long as it occurs within certain parameters. Clinical variations can be either warranted or unwarranted. Warranted clinical variation is essentially unavoidable, as all doctors, nurses, and other practitioners have a different understanding or insight into a particular problem and utilize different protocols of problem management. On the other hand, unwarranted clinical variation is about the overuse or underuse of certain therapies, treatments, or diagnosis materials in a way that potentially hurts patient outcomes or the sustainability of the health system. The second type of variation is much more problematic in healthcare practice because it can increase the vulnerability to errors [11].

4. Sources of variation

The major sources of variation can be grouped into two major classes: common cause variation also called random variation which can happen in stable processes and special cause variation which is mainly seen in unstable processes. Both types will be explained later.

5. Contributing factors of the variability of health care

The variability in clinical care practice often stems from two separate issues [12]:

1. *Operational variability* refers to differences in care delivered directly by different involved in the patient care process. While each provider delivers care based on his/her understanding of the patient's diagnosis and treatment plan, this can lead to significant differences in the way of delivering patient care.

2. *Knowledge variability* refers to differences in expertise among medical staff. This type of variability is often difficult to assess because it's based on an individual provider's educational and experience level.

In this chapter, we will try to highlight the top-quality improvement initiatives that have significant roles in standardizing healthcare processes, reducing variation in clinical practice, and achieving predictable results, for patients, healthcare systems, and organizations. These initiatives include:

1. Clinical practice guidelines and pathways

2. Policies and procedures (P&Ps)

3. Data-driven performance

4. The 5S methodology

5. High 5s project

6. Clinical audit

7. Quality of thinking

8. Education and training

9. Accreditation process

10. Care bundles

6. Clinical practice guidelines and pathways

6.1 Background

Clinical practice guidelines (CPGs) and integrated care pathways (ICPs) play a vital role in modern healthcare by providing a framework for standardizing medical practices and improving the quality and safety of patient care. These evidence-based tools offer healthcare professionals a structured approach to clinical decision-making, ensuring that patients receive the most effective and appropriate care. This article explores the significance of CPGs and ICPs in enhancing healthcare outcomes, quality improvement, and patient safety.

Clinical practice guidelines (CPGs) are systematically developed, evidence-based recommendations and statements that guide healthcare professionals in making informed decisions about the most appropriate healthcare interventions for specific clinical situations or conditions. CPGs are typically founded on a comprehensive review of the best available medical evidence, expert consensus, and the consideration of patient values and preferences. They aim to standardize and improve the quality of healthcare by providing a structured framework for clinical decision-making, diagnosis, treatment, and patient management [13].

Integrated care pathways (ICPs), also referred to as care pathways or clinical pathways, are multidisciplinary plans of care that outline the essential steps, activities, and interventions required for the effective management of patients with specific medical conditions, across the entire continuum of care. ICPs are designed to promote collaboration among healthcare professionals from various disciplines and ensure a seamless and coordinated delivery of care. They often incorporate CPGs and evidence-based practices into a structured framework that helps optimize patient outcomes, streamline healthcare processes, and enhance patient and caregiver engagement. They are also considered one of the main types of CPG implementation tools [14, 15]. ICPs are particularly valuable for managing complex or chronic conditions by outlining the most appropriate care trajectories and facilitating communication and continuity of care among healthcare providers.

6.2 Evidence-based medicine and CPGs

Evidence-based medicine (EBM) is of paramount importance in healthcare as it ensures that clinical decisions and interventions are grounded in the best available scientific evidence. EBM promotes the rational, efficient, and patient-centered delivery of care by systematically integrating rigorous research findings with clinical expertise and patient values and preferences. It enhances the quality and safety of healthcare, reducing variations in practice and minimizing the potential for risk or harm. By adhering to EBM principles, healthcare professionals can optimize diagnostic accuracy, and treatment outcomes, reduce unnecessary interventions, and allocate resources more effectively, ultimately leading to improved patient outcomes, increased patient satisfaction, and the continuous advancement of medical knowledge and practice [13].

EBM forms the foundation of contemporary and modern healthcare. CPGs and ICPs are essential tools to apply EBM and Evidence-Based Healthcare in general, as they translate the latest research findings into practical recommendations for clinical practice and serve as a bridge between research and patient care.

One of the primary roles of CPGs and ICPs is to standardize care across healthcare settings which in turn leads to greater consistency, integration, and predictability in healthcare delivery. When healthcare professionals follow established CPGs and ICPs, patients can expect a uniform level of care, reducing variations and the potential for errors. This standardization is particularly critical in complex and high-risk areas, such as surgery and critical care.

6.3 Improving quality and safety of care

Adherence to CPGs and ICPs can significantly enhance the quality of care provided to patients [16, 17]. By following evidence-based recommendations, healthcare providers can optimize treatment plans, reduce complications, and achieve better patient outcomes. CPGs help identify best practices, allowing healthcare institutions to measure and improve their performance continuously.

Patient safety is a paramount concern in healthcare, and CPGs and ICPs contribute significantly to minimizing risks. CPGs have a significant role in aiding the identification and mitigation of potential errors and adverse events [15, 18]. They guide infection control, medication management, and other critical aspects of patient safety, ultimately reducing the likelihood of harm.

Moreover, by promoting efficient and effective care, these tools can lead to cost savings for healthcare systems that further highlight the economic benefits of using CPGs and ICPs. Standardized approaches reduce unnecessary procedures, hospital readmissions, and complications, resulting in better resource allocation and improved cost-effectiveness.

6.4 Challenges in guideline and pathway implementation

Implementing CPGs and their ICPs in healthcare settings faces several challenges [15, 18, 19]. The complexity of CPGs, varying levels of the quality of evidence, and the need for adaptation to local contexts (i.e., contextualization) can hinder effective implementation. Additionally, healthcare professionals may experience information overload, leading to difficulty in staying updated with numerous CPGs for the same health topics. Barriers to adoption include resistance to change, lack of awareness, and limited time and resources. Strategies to overcome these barriers involve engaging all relevant stakeholders in CPG development or adaptation, providing regular training, involving quality and clinical champions, regular audits and feedback, involving patients, and integrating CPGs into clinical workflows and ICPs. Successful models, such as the use of electronic health records for CPG dissemination and clinical decision support through automation or digitalization of CPGs and ICPs, have shown positive impacts on patient care by improving adherence to evidence-based practices.

6.5 Future, innovations, and the way forward

The landscape of CPGs and ICPs is evolving with advances in technology and methodology. As healthcare moves toward more dynamic, real-time decision-making, the development and dissemination of CPGs are increasingly incorporating sophisticated data analysis and digital platforms. This evolution is aimed at ensuring that guidelines are current, evidence-based, and readily accessible to healthcare professionals, especially with emerging concepts like living CPGs, living systematic reviews, and living sphere evidence [17].

Emerging technologies, such as machine learning and natural language processing, are revolutionizing the way CPGs are developed and disseminated. These technologies facilitate the analysis of large datasets to identify patterns and trends, which can inform CPG development. Additionally, digital dissemination platforms, including mobile apps and online portals, are making it easier for healthcare providers to access and apply guidelines in clinical practice.

The integration of artificial intelligence (AI) and data analytics is expected to pave the way for personalized CPG recommendations. AI algorithms can analyze patient data, consider individual health conditions and preferences, and suggest customized care plans and pathways. This approach aims to enhance the precision of treatments, improve patient outcomes, and streamline clinical decision-making processes, ushering in a new era of personalized medicine in CPG implementation.

7. Policies and Procedures (P&Ps)

7.1 Background

Policies are defined by the Joint Commission International (JCI) as rules and principles that guide and inform the organization's procedures and processes whereas a procedure is defined as step-by-step instructions for how a task is performed [20]. Delivery of high-quality healthcare services requires up-to-date policies and procedures that reflect the latest good practice, and ensure compliance with the regulatory and legislative requirements [21]. In addition to their role in facilitating adherence to healthcare laws, accreditation requirements, licensing, and certification standards, clinical teams including doctors, nurses, pharmacists, and other care providers who are involved in patient care, P&Ps can play a vital role in communicating expectations and standards to staff, set guidelines for day-to-day operations and improvements, streamline processes and enhance patient safety [22].

7.2 Why policies and procedures are important?

Policies and procedures are essential components of effective quality improvement and patient safety programs for the following reasons:

1. Assist in carrying out daily patient care by clarifying the roles and responsibilities.

2. Serve as a unique communication tool between the treatment team.

3. Unify the practices between multidisciplinary teams and reduce the potential error rate that could happen due to variations in clinical practice.

4. Improve consistency and accuracy of the clinical process.

5. Guide decision-making process.

6. Protect the organization's reputation and minimize any potential liabilities.

7. Improve confidence and satisfaction in teamwork.

7.3 General guidance for writing effective P&Ps

All policies and procedures should be written in simple and clear language to make them comprehensible to everyone. Minimize using abbreviations that could interrupt or confuse the reader. It is recommended to avoid using complex sentences with multiple clauses that would complicate understanding what the policy is about. They also must state clearly who does what and articulate the roles and responsibilities of individuals and departments responsible for carrying out certain duties. Finally, all P&Ps should be accessible to all teams.

7.4 Types of healthcare P&Ps

Healthcare P&Ps can be divided into five major types [23]:

1. *Patient care:* is related to all P&Ps that guide clinicians to perform daily and routine patient care operations in the healthcare practice.

2. *Health and safety:* any kind of policy that helps staff deal with and handle any safety and health risks that could arise during patient care.

3. *Drug handling and management:* all types of policies and guidelines that assist in handling the medication management cycle transfer, storage, prescribing, preparation, administration, and so on.

4. *Information management:* all policies that support proper management of sensitive information inside healthcare facilities. They can include topics such as confidentiality, security, privacy, integrity of information, and distribution of medical records. It also includes retention time for patient medical records and other information

5. *Administrative and human resources:* it pertains to all policies that deal with recruitment, retention, development, and continuing education of staff.

7.5 Management of P&Ps

Policies and procedures must be developed through a standardized and systematic process starting by addressing the need for them that could stem from new legal requirements, and then assembling a multidisciplinary team (owners) that will be responsible for drafting, reviewing, finalizing, and approving the policy.

Before implementing the P&PSs, the staff should be familiar with them and this can be achieved through focused training. Adherence of the staff should be monitored and any challenges or obstacles during implementation should be raised and fixed by the quality improvement team. Policies and procedures must be reviewed and updated periodically to ensure their relevancy and effectiveness.

8. Data-driven performance

8.1 Background

Data is a vital and valuable resource in healthcare, it is like a compass or the dashboard of the vehicle that serves to monitor its performance and alert the driver of any problem. In the healthcare field, we use Key Performance Indicators (KPIs) to track the improvement process (observe, analyze, optimize, and transform a healthcare process) and to make sure that staff are adhering to the standards of care. These metrics also can be used to compare (benchmarking) the organization's performance to other similar healthcare facilities and identify areas for improvement [24]. Furthermore, they can help to support the effectiveness and efficiency of clinical care as well as to enhance continuous performance measurement [25]. Finally, these metrics can enable informed decision-making based on actual healthcare delivery models, for example, healthcare practitioners and leaders can use accurate, valid, reliable, timely, relevant, legible, and complete data to proactively adjust the clinical course of treatment for individual patients [26, 27]. Performance indicators should not be seen as a quality improvement tool that will provide feasible solutions for how to fix the performance problems, they act only as diagnostic means and trigger the organization for any deviation in their process's performance.

8.2 Sources of data

There are many sources for getting data either internal sources within the healthcare facility or external from accreditation, government, semi-government, non-profit patient advocacy, and commercial organizations in the field. The data collected from internal sources assist in regularly evaluating the performance of healthcare processes whereas the data used from external sources facilitate comparison with other organizations in the same field and have a similar scope of services as well as assist in setting performance targets. **Table 1** shows the main sources of data.

8.3 Performance indicators

Performance monitoring is a continuous process that involves collecting data to determine if a service is meeting desired standards or targets [27]. Key Performance Indicators (KPIs) are well-defined performance measures that are used to observe, analyze, optimize, and transform a healthcare process to increase satisfaction for both patients and healthcare providers alike. These metrics are commonly used by care facilities to compare their performance to other care facilities and identify areas for improvement [24]. The performance measures are formulated either based on standards determined through evidence-based academic literature or the consensus of experts when evidence is unavailable [27].

Internal sources	External sources
• Occurrence reports/summaries • Ongoing quality measurement • Surveys, interviews, questionnaires • Direct observation (clinical audit, walkarounds) • Clinical records, reports/profiles (pharmacy, lab, blood bank, etc.) • Infection control reports • Regulatory and accreditation reports • Clinical review findings • Incident reporting system	• National registry reports • Communicable Disease Control (CDC) reports • Research projects/literature (e.g., MEDLINE) • Clinical protocols, guidelines, and practice parameters (medical colleges and boards) • National Guideline Clearinghouse • International library of measure • Accreditation bodies reports

Table 1.
Source of data.

8.4 Type of performance indicators

According to the Donabedian model, performance indicators are divided into three types structure, process, and outcome:

1. *Structure measure*: it evaluates the context in which healthcare is delivered from two aspects: the capacity of the physical settings (buildings, staff number, cost per unit, and used equipment, medicines, and systems) and the capabilities of care providers (staff qualifications, training, and competencies).

2. *Process measure*: it reflects the way health systems and processes work to deliver the desired outcome by applying specific actions that are consistent with professional standards of care and evidence-based guidelines for diagnosis.

3. *Outcome measure:* it refers to the effects or the outcome of healthcare such as reduced morbidity and mortality, reduced length of stay, reduced hospital-acquired infections, adverse incidents or harm.

8.5 Balancing measure

Balancing measure is another type of measure that aims to look at a system from different directions/dimensions. Any changes designed to improve one part of the system should not cause new problems in other parts of the system. For example, for reducing the time patients spend on a ventilator after surgery we must make sure that the reintubation rates are not increasing.

8.6 What is a benchmark?

Benchmark refers to a point of reference that is used to evaluate the performance or quality of something. It is a standard or a set of criteria against which something can be measured or compared [28]. Benchmarking can be conducted internally by comparing the performance of specific processes with similar processes in different

Common cause variation	Special cause variation
Caused by natural or ordinary causes	Caused by non-ordinary and unnatural causes
Inherent to system or process.	Non-inherent to the process design.
Predictable	Unpredictable
Affects all the outcomes of a process	Affects some but not necessarily all aspects of the process.
Result in a stable process	Result in unstable process
develop and test ideas that might result in improvements to the process and system.	Require investigation of the underlying causes of variations and take correct actions to fix it.

Source: ©2023 Institute for Healthcare Improvement. Used with permission.

Table 2.
Types of process variations.

areas of the same organization. For example, comparing ventilator-associated pneumonia (VAP) rates in different medical intensive care units (ICUs). It can be done also externally (locally, nationally, or internationally); within healthcare organizations of similar size and scope, against medical practice literature, or through participation in national or international databases. Whether internal or external benchmarking the ultimate aim is to provide clinicians with valuable information that guides them in the decision-making process.

8.7 Process variation

Variation refers to the lack of uniformity and difference in the performance of the process compared to the acceptable performance of peers. In clinical practice, clinical variation can drive poor care quality, wasted resources, and lead to excessive cost of services [29].

8.8 Types of process variations

There are two types of process variations common cause variation and special cause variation. **Table 2** shows the main differences between them [30].

9. 5S methodology

9.1 Background

The 5S methodology is identified as one of the most common lean management tools used not only to improve the workplace environment but also to improve the functional aspects of the process. 5S was developed in Japan and used by Toyota [31]. The 5S methodology is also called lean and it is composed of five Japanese words Seiri, Seiton, Seiso, Seiketsu, and Shitsuke, which means sort, set in order, shine, standardize, and sustain. 5S methodology is a set of actions that need to be conducted systematically in a sequence order one after the other with the full participation of staff responsible for the process and it should be repeated continuously [32]. The 5S methodology can benefit any organization that is genuinely committed to becoming less

Japanese	English	What is it about?
Seiri	Sort	Eliminate unnecessary items and tools from the workplace area.
Seiton	Set	Arranging items in the workplace area logically and efficiently.
Seiso	Shine	Clean the workplace area to maintain a safe environment.
Seiketsu	Standardize	Standardize the best practices in the workplace area right after implementing the first 3S.
Shitsuke	Sustain	Make the already-developed processes part of the practitioner's daily routine (self-discipline).

Table 3.
General principles of 5S methodology.

wasteful, more efficient, and keen on enhancing safety, establishing goals, and streamlining the workflow of the process [33]. **Table 3** shows the general principles of 5S.

To facilitate the application of 5S and avoid fall back of the first 3S and consequently long-term implementation for the whole methodology, it is recommended to divide it into two phases, the initial phase focuses on the achievement of the first 3S (Sort, Set, and Shine), and the second phase focuses on the last 2S (Standardize and Sustain) [32]. In the context of healthcare quality improvement, the 5S methodology has been recognized as one of the lean-quality improvement tools and it was used to maximize added value by removing all unnecessary factors that do not generate value [34]. The method had a great impact on the promoting of healthcare services effectively, and increased staff motivation in healthcare facilities where resources are scarce and prevailing of other demotivating factors [35, 36]. On the other hand, applying 5S can enhance patient safety by reducing the rate of errors, improving the efficiency of healthcare services, reducing waiting time, and creating a safer and more organized environment for patient care.

9.2 Scope of using 5S in healthcare practice

The 5S methodology can be applied widely in healthcare practice. It can be used, for example, in the following areas:

1. *Error reporting systems*: implementing robust systems for reporting and tracking errors, near misses, and adverse events can help identify potential risks and prevent future occurrences.

2. *Medication reconciliation*: developing thorough processes for reconciling a patient's medication history is essential to avoid adverse drug events and ensure accurate and safe medication administration.

3. *Fall prevention programs:* implementing protocols to assess and minimize fall risks for patients, especially those with mobility issues, can prevent injuries and improve safety.

4. *Standardized protocols*: developing standardized protocols for various procedures and care processes, such as surgical checklists and hand hygiene protocols, can improve consistency and reduce errors.

5. *Patient identification protocols*: implementing strict protocols for patient identification, especially before administering medications or performing any procedures, can mitigate the risk of errors.

9.3 Example for applying the 5S in healthcare practice

The 5S methodology can be applied in clinical areas as follows:

1. *Sort*: this involves removing unnecessary items from the clinical and operational areas in the hospitals to eliminate clutter and improve efficiency. In healthcare settings, this can help ensure that essential patient care items are easily accessible while reducing the risk of errors caused by confusion or clutter, putting in consideration removing the extra unnecessary equipment and supplies will decrease the chance of mistakes in utilizing the wrong supplies.

2. *Set in order*: in patient care areas, this can involve organizing medical supplies and equipment in a standardized and consistent manner, making it easier for healthcare providers to find what they need quickly and reducing the potential for error.

3. *Shine:* in healthcare, this *S* is a crucial part of infection control programs. By maintaining a clean and safe environment, the risk of patient harm due to contaminated surfaces or equipment will be reduced. If the clinical area is carefully inspected and all old notices, posters, broken equipment, and unused machines are removed from the area, the potential hazards and risks can be identified easily [37]. Shining can be expanded to include cleaning all types of equipment that are under use like computers, keyboards, monitors, tables, etc. Cleaning should be conducted periodically with the full participation of all the staff in the area. Using a simple cleaning checklist can improve the execution of this phase as well as assist the CQI and the infection control department in the tracing process [32].

4. *Standardize:* after implementing the first three 3S's, the next step is to standardize care processes to ensure the consistency and reliability of the care provided to patients. This S involves creating standardized protocols for handling daily clinical tasks such as medication administration process, patient handoffs, prevention of patient falls, and other critical care processes to minimize any potential for errors and harm.

5. *Sustain:* this may involve ongoing training, regular audits, and continuous improvement efforts to ensure that patient safety remains a top priority. To ensure this phase, it is recommended to link this S with a group of Key performance measures, in which any trend or special variation can be triggered quickly.

10. The high 5S project

10.1 Background

Without a doubt, patient safety has gained considerable global attention and focus from health leaders, researchers, healthcare providers, and business and management development organizations. It is a fundamental principle of high-quality patient care [38]. The safety of patients has been incorporated into many healthcare delivery models developed by various healthcare organizations, for example, is a key component of the Institute of Medicine's (IOM) six domains of healthcare quality, which are abbreviated as STEEEP (Safe, Timely, Effective, Efficient, Equitable, and Patient-centered).

Furthermore, it is one of the key indicators and measures used to assess the safety of healthcare practices. Patient safety is defined by the World Health Organization (WHO) as the absence of preventable harm to a patient and the reduction of risk of unnecessary harm associated with health care to an acceptable minimum [39]. Within the context of a broader health system, patient safety is a framework of organized activities that creates cultures, processes, procedures, behaviors, technologies, and environments in health care that consistently and sustainably lower risks, reduce the occurrence of avoidable harm, make the error less likely and reduce the impact of harm when it does occur [39]. The WHO had declared and adopted several important patient safety initiatives, to urge and guide member states, particularly in low- and middle-income countries with fragile health systems to focus and prioritize patient safety as one of the most important components of healthcare delivery through publications, capacity building, education, campaigns, tools, and relevant conferences [40].

Clean Hand is Safer Care, Safe Surgery Saves Lives (surgical safety checklist), Patient Safety research, anti-microbial Resistance, and the multi-professional patient safety curriculum guide, Global Patient Safety Collaborative (GPSC), and Medication without Harm are among the WHO global Patient safety initiatives [40]. The 5 s project was another WHO patient safety initiative, and it will be the focus of this section.

10.2 What is the high 5s project?

The high 5s project is one of the important global patient safety initiatives that was launched by the World Health Organization (WHO) in 2006. It aims to address continuing major concerns about patient safety around the world as well as to facilitate the implementation and evaluation of standardized patient safety solutions within a global learning community to achieve measurable, significant, and sustainable reductions in challenging patient safety problems [41].

10.3 Scope of the 5s project

The five major components of the High 5s project are:

1. Develop and implement Standardized Operating Protocols (SOPs)

2. Create an impact evaluation strategy.

3. Collect, report, and analyze validated data.

4. Develop a collaborative learning community.

5. Disseminating learned lessons globally.

There are five SOPs and associated evaluation instruments were developed between 2007 and 2009 to address the following challenges: Medication Accuracy at

Transitions in Care, Correct Procedure at the Correct Body Site, Use of Concentrated Injectable Medicines, Communication During Patient Care Handovers, and Health Care-Associated Infections [42].

10.4 Attributes of the high 5s project

There are two unique features of the high 5s project which are [42]:

1. *Standardization* is the process of developing, agreeing upon, and implementing technical or uniform specifications, criteria, methods, processes, designs, or practices that can increase compatibility, interoperability, safety, repeatability, and quality. Process standardization is the specification and communication of a process at a level of detail sufficient to permit consistent and verifiable implementation by different users at different times and in different settings. Standardization can reduce variation and minimize the tendency of process failure. It also enables shared learning, facilitates multi-disciplinary teamwork, and improves efficiency in interactions by establishing optimum conditions.

2. *Evaluation:* the high 5s project evaluation approach addresses the impact measurement challenge from different perspectives, including qualitative data collection regarding the SOP implementation experiences, quantitative performance measurement results, event analysis, and organization culture assessment. These methods were used to assess the feasibility and impact of implementing standardized patient safety protocols.

11. Clinical audit

11.1 Background

Audit is a Latin word that means to hear [43]. Clinical audit was defined by the National Institute for Health and Clinical Excellence (NICE) as a quality improvement process that seeks to improve patient care and outcomes through a systematic review against explicit criteria and the implementation of change [44]. It is also defined as a process that seeks to identify where improvements can be made within healthcare services by measuring them against evidence-based standards [45].

11.2 Audit vs. quality improvement

As we mentioned before in this chapter, quality improvement (QI) is a systematic approach that is used to study whole processes (clinical and non-clinical) formulating healthcare systems unlike clinical audit it is mainly clinically oriented. Although the auditing process is quite longer than some quality improvement approaches like PDSA and it can take months till completed, both tools have the same goal which is to look at the current status of healthcare standards and think how they could be improved. On the other hand, the scope of the audit is broader than QI approaches, it can be conducted on a small scale, for example, auditing a specific process in the hospital, or auditing the whole level of care (Primary Care, Home Care, and a group of Hospitals (trust) and or it can be carried out at national level (national clinical audits).

11.3 What is clinical audit

The audit is one of the key quality improvement measures as well as one of the main pillars of clinical governance and it allows healthcare organizations to continually work toward improving the quality of care and optimizing patient safety by showing them where they are falling short allowing them to implement the required improvements and repeat the cycle to assess the effectiveness of implemented change [46]. The main goal of clinical audits is to facilitate the process of quality improvement because that will be very beneficial and will lead to improved outcomes for patients. Clinical audits can look at care at a national level (national clinical audits) and local clinical audits can also be carried out locally in trusts, hospitals, or primary care practices wherever healthcare is provided.

11.4 The cycle of clinical audit

There are six stages of the commonly accepted audit cycle, and each stage is detailed as follows [46]:

1. *Choose the audit topic* (identify problem) for example, patients waiting too long in accident and emergency (A&E).

2. *Defining standards/criteria*, for example, guidelines recommend that 95% of patients should wait <4 hours.

3. *Collect data*, for example, record over a week how long patients wait (determining that 92% wait for <4 h).

4. *Analysis*, for example, 92% versus 95% target, areas for improvement.

5. *Implementing change*, for example, an action plan to help reach the target.

6. *Reaudit*, for example, do steps 1–5 again until reaching the target then set the required measures to sustain gained change.

11.5 Audit vs. research

Clinical audit and research can overlap with each other in clinical practice and it is very important to recognize the differences between them. **Table 4** explores the key differences between these two tools:

11.6 Barriers and enablers factors for effective audit

There are many factors that can influence for conducting a good audit, these include lack of expertise, inadequate data due to lack of documentation or record keeping, auditing being conducted subjectively and not based on proven standards, lack of leadership support, and scarcity of resources due to limited budgets. Quality of feedback also can limit the benefits of the change that would be brought from the audit. In contrast, performing an effective audit requires training, allocating the time for the staff, and having a reliable source of data like electronic health records, an information technology system that bridges the gap between routine collected data and auditing as well as the independence of the clinical auditor.

Clinical audit	Research
It is a continuous cycle of improvement	It is a systematic study
It aims to: • Measures the effectiveness of health care against agreed and proven standards of care for high quality. • Take the corrective actions to align the practice with these standards. • Implement, monitor, and sustain the changes when indicated.	It aims to: • Answer and analyze various questions and occurrences in the field of science. • Develop hypotheses and test their validity. • Enhance the quality of care by producing knowledge on what constitutes best practice to inform the guidelines
Tell us where we are doing it.	Discover what should doing

Table 4.
Key differences between clinical audit and research.

12. Quality of thinking

One of the quality definitions is doing the right thing right. However, the right thing is not determined by quality per se but on a higher level like strategic planning may be doing our tasks right and free of flaws or harm. Healthcare services can extend beyond just being safe care to be timely, effective, efficient, equitable, and patient-centered.

Therefore, safety is the number one priority as the patient should not add more negative health issues than what they already have. Additionally, they need to be treated for what they came for promptly, with an effective outcome in an efficient way with the same rights as others and in a nice way. This could be summarized also in three words devised by IHI (Institute of Healthcare Improvement): be nice to me, treat me, and do not harm me **Figure 1**. For this to be achieved there are four factors at play affecting these dimensions causing less quality of care.

There are four factors of system thinking Patient, Provider, Environment, and Task, and since we are using an acronym, we might call it PPET for short, **Figure 2**.

Much work has been put into the environmental factor (sometimes called system or facility and here it includes all the surroundings from equipment, devices, lights, flooring, policy & and procedures, pathways, and protocols) as it is believed it will fail the provider from doing their task right and this is true but proved inadequate as error rates are on the increase.

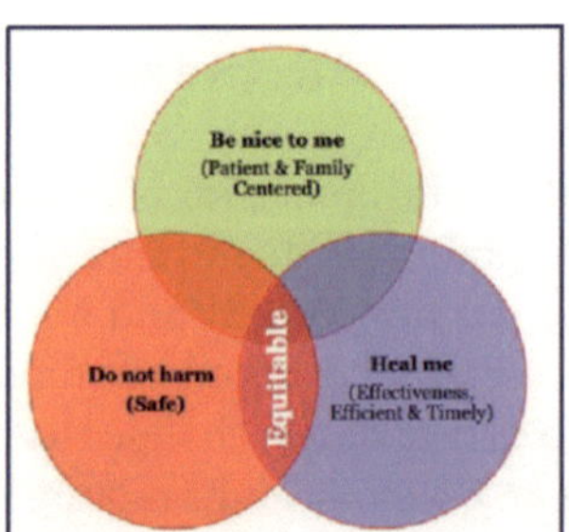

Figure 1.
The IHI three principles of care.

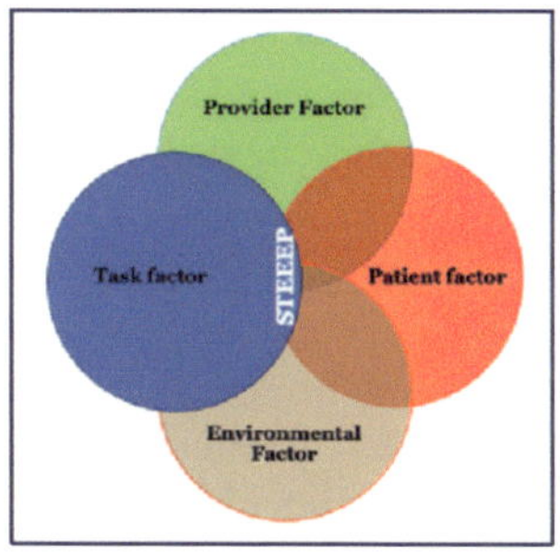

Figure 2.
Four components of quality thinking.

The patient factor could be out of this chapter's scope as it needs a complete chapter on how to communicate well with patients and get the complete information enabling providers to achieve and reach a proper diagnosis for example.

Task factor is also another important factor where different tasks require different and higher demands of awareness and mindfulness as in the case of the rule-based and knowledge-based tasks compared with skill or routine-based tasks. However, the most important factor that had little attention is the provider factor. Providers could unintentionally fail to perform their tasks appropriately leading to system failure and undesirable patient outcomes. Here we want to talk about the quality of the provider's thinking in achieving the dimension of Quality STEEEP (Safe, Timely, Effective, Efficient, Equitable, and Patient-centered).

One would agree that the same task can be done differently by different providers and even it can be done with variations by the same provider. The same task can be done incorrectly by certain providers but may be not done by others. Similarly, some providers will make errors with patients and even not follow the policy and procedure of the system.

The quality of work or performance is linked and affected by the provider's thinking styles, personality traits, emotional intelligence (EI), and many other intangible factors like sub-clinical psychopathy when it comes to counterproductive behavior at the workplace which would compromise patient safety. Therefore, maybe we need to come up with a new terminology like human internal and external factors to be more specific so the external factors cover everything outside the provider (e.g., system, environment, policy & and procedures, patients, tasks, protocols, clinical pathways, etc.) and internal factors which are intrinsic or brain structure and makeup of individuals that process internally everything external and produce certain behavior accordingly.

Organizations should start taking this aspect seriously to understand the variations among healthcare providers and even within the same service providers to understand why they behave in certain ways that might expose them to more patient safety errors and even counterproductive work behavior. For example, the style of thinking in terms of experiential style (ES, more associated with effect and rapid response) and rational style (RS, more conscious and analytical) were found to differ between nurses and physicians. Nurses relied significantly more on ES compared to physicians and one positive aspect of this is that higher individual scores in ES would report errors compared to lower ES. However, higher scores in RS were shown to be linked to lower error rates, but it is better if the individual had higher scores in both RS and ES to have a real positive effect on lowering clinical errors [47].

Another intrinsic factor that affects the quality of work is EI which has many dimensions. For example, creative thinking was linked to the Sociability factor of the EI, the higher the score the more creative the person is. Additionally, these factors also affected the error rate in the person [48]. Another EI dimension that has a positive impact on the quality of care is self-control where higher scores had significantly safer quality of care [49].

On the negative side, lower scores in EI are associated with self-harm, and personality disorders that might be harmful to patient safety [49].

Personality traits were shown to predict which individual might be at higher risk of erring, have negative qualities in the workplace like bullying, and even how they would care for patient's needs. Higher scores in the personality trait of Conscientiousness would lower the risk of clinical errors and in pharmacy staff this had a positive effect on how pharmacy staff would recommend treatments that are less likely to cause pain or interfere with the patient's daily activities hence enhancing safer care and better quality of patient experience [50].

Agreeableness personality trait had also a positive impact on the quality of care if the individual had higher scores, however, it has a detrimental effect on the quality of care from an error rate point of view and provider-patient communication if the score is low and also it makes the individual at a significantly higher risk of initiation of bullying and violence. In general individuals with high scores of agreeableness were found to be friendly, cooperative, and supportive whereas individuals with low scores tended to be selfish and less caring. Additionally, high scores in neuroticism were associated with violence, more anxiety, a higher risk of burnout, and errors [49].

One of the explanations for certain personality traits and EI individuals being more at risk of lower quality of care from an error point of view, bullying, violence, less cooperation, and shorter span of attention could be because they tend to be more anxious than others [51]. Healthcare is a stressful environment of long hours, less time for proper meals, burnout, lack of sleep, and stressful demands for problem resolution and patients' needs. With more anxiety as a normal base for these individuals then they would feel the stress of work even much more than others. Stress like this was shown to be associated with a negative effect on the hippocampus and the amygdala affecting their volume which in turn affects memory, learning, and accessing information they would be much more emotional and would be caught in a vicious circle leading them to errors and negative workplace behaviors [52–54].

In conclusion, quality of work depends on external and internal factors surrounding the provider which put them at more risk of errors and other negative behavior. Healthcare organizations must have a holistic approach to quality of care if they want to reduce harm to patients, staff, and the organization.

13. Education and training

13.1 Background

Training is important in health and social care, to ensure safety for everyone involved in delivering care and for those receiving it and to maintain the highest levels of care quality [55]. Quality improvement training programs were defined as any activity that explicitly aimed to teach professionals about methods that could be used to analyze and improve the quality of healthcare. In recent years, these programs have grown fast to include ongoing education like workshops, online courses, collaboratives, and ad hoc training set up to support running specific improvement projects. This growth in the quality training programs has supported the participants in improving their knowledge, skills, and attitudes and utilizing what they have learned in their clinical practice [56]. Education and training can break down barriers to providing safe care, creating an environment where all staff learn from error, patients are at the center of care, treated with openness and honesty, and where staff are trained to focus on patient needs [57]. Quality training programs can also assist practitioners in complying with local and national required standards, policies, and practice guidelines and ultimately unifying the protocols of care.

13.2 How to develop an effective training program?

Developing effective training programs on quality and patient safety requirements can begin with assessing the existing training needs (gaps: current training and those required to meet the goal) and this can be done by gathering data from various sources in the hospital followed by developing the training programs based on the findings of gap analyses. The source of data includes but is not limited to:

- Key Performance Indicators (KPIs) reports
- Incident reporting system
- Root Cause Analysis (RCA) recommendations
- Accreditation body findings
- Recommendation of quality improvement projects
- Tracing and auditing reports
- Patient safety walk-rounds
- Failure Mode and Effect Analysis (FMEA) recommendations

Table 5 shows some examples of these training programs and their benefits for the healthcare practitioner.

13.3 Evaluation of training and education process

Training evaluation is an essential component of capacity-building initiatives. It helps to assess the effectiveness of the training program, identifies areas of improvement, and ensures that the training meets the needs of the participants and that invested resources in training are being used effectively [57].

Evaluation can be done by one of the evaluation methods such as pre-and post-training assessments, Kirkpatrick's Four Levels of Evaluation, CIPP (Context, Input, Process, Product) model, observation, Surveys, and Questionnaires, or any other alternative method that is approved by the organization's education training department [58].

#	Education	Benefit
1	Data Management Process	It enables the trainer to understand the whole data management process including collection, validation, and analysis as well as tracking the process performance over time and picking up any deviations.
2	Auditing and Tracing Methodologies	It helps the trainer monitor the adherence of clinicians to the required standards, guidelines, and policies.
3	Performance Improvement Approaches	It assists the trainer in leading the improvement journey by utilizing the right quality improvement tools.
4	Risk Management Approaches	Whether is a proactive approach like Failure Mode and Effect Analysis (FMEA) or reactive ones like Root Cause Analysis (RCA), the trainer will be capable of forecasting any potential failure that could happen and any actual failures already occurred and setting the appropriate risk reduction solutions
5	Standards of Care Requirements	It provides the trainer with knowledge and skills about the required patient care standards and how to meet them through policies, procedures, and clinical practice guidelines.

Table 5.
Quality training programs.

14. Accreditation process

14.1 Background

Accreditation is about turning the noise of the complex health system into musical rhythms. According to the International Society for Quality in Healthcare, accreditation is a process "in which trained external peer reviewers evaluate a healthcare organization's compliance with pre-established performance standards [59]. In other words, it's an approval seal to show to what extent healthcare organizations are committed to providing safe patient care. Being accredited means the organization has met the highest and most excellent standards of care. The Joint Commission International (JCI) defines a standard as a statement that defines the performance expectations, structures, or processes that must be in place for an organization to provide safe and high-quality patient care, treatment, and services [20]. Standards also are described as the minimum level as the minimum accepted level of practice and quality. They are also developed in alignment with regulatory requirements, ensuring that healthcare facilities conform to laws and regulations related to patient safety. Examples include that healthcare facilities are required to report any medical equipment-related incidents to the National Food & Drug Authority, and healthcare providers are not allowed to practice their professions unless the relevant national regulatory entities license them. A quality management system (QMS), on the other hand, is a mechanism to ensure that procedures are being carried out in line with agreed standards and full participation by all staff members [59].

14.2 Accreditation vs. regulations

These two concepts are not identical. Accreditation as mentioned before is an approval seal to show to what extent the healthcare organizations are committed to providing safe patient care and it is granted by an independent accrediting body that the organization has met applicable standards and requirements, while regulations are group of rules that strictly followed, and they enforced by national authorities and regulators like Ministries of Health, Medical and Nursing counsels, Food Drug Authorities, etc.

14.3 What are the benefits of accreditation?

Despite the accreditation process emphasizing how healthcare organizations adhere to applicable standards, the ultimate goal is how continuously improve the healthcare system and processes. The accreditation can assist the health organizations in:

1. Building up the quality management system (QMS) with required policies, protocols, procedures, and checklists.

2. Assist in building a quality measurement database.

3. Provide effective comparison with self, and others as well as with best practice.

4. Assisting the organization in developing and disseminating a culture of continuous improvement for all staff.

5. Ensure a safe care environment by reducing the potential risks that could jeopardize care recipients and caregivers alike.

6. Establish an organizational culture of openness, and transparency, speak up, and learn from past experiences that facilitate improvement initiatives and sustain change.

7. Assist in Reducing the variations in the clinical practice that could put patient safety at big risk.

8. Improve the outcomes of healthcare services.

9. Provide a comprehensive framework for healthcare organizations to enhance patient safety by incorporating best evidence-based practice.

14.4 Accreditation cycle

The accreditation preparation cycle consists of five phases: the first phase is planning which is about conducting a gap analysis of the current situation to see what the required documents (what we already have and what we should have). After identifying the gaps, the next step is to assemble multiple teams to prepare the required documentation. Then the next phase is to educate and train staff about the required documents. After that, monitor the compliance of the staff with required documents by conducting unplanned periodic audits. This cycle should be repeated until reaching the optimum level of performance. Once the optimum level of performance has been achieved, the final phase is to maintain this level of practice. Continuous leadership support, in place-equipped, quality management system, staff vigilance, and commitment are the key drivers to sustain the gain change.

14.5 Standards of patient care

Standards of patient care are those standards related to direct patient-family care. These standards can vary from one accreditor to another. Below are some examples of them:

1. Patient care (access, assessment, transition, and continuity of care)

2. Patient safety

3. Medication management

4. Infection control and prevention

5. Anesthesia and surgical

All standards including the care standards are developed with input and information from various sources that include [60]:

1. Health care organizations

2. Subject matter experts

3. Scientific literature and industry guidelines

4. Technical Advisory Panels

5. Other key stakeholders

15. Care bundles

15.1 Background

The concept of care bundles has been developed in 2001 by the Institute for Healthcare Improvement (IHI). A bundle is defined as a set of evidence-based practices—generally three to five—that when performed collectively and reliably, have been proven to improve patient outcomes [61, 62]. The Bundle of care is an ongoing process that's repeated daily until the patient no longer requires an invasive device or his or her status has improved. All of the elements of the bundle must be performed in a sequence of series of steps by one healthcare team within the same time frame to ensure that clinical improvement occurs. The adoption of 'care bundles' can be seen as a fundamental shift in thinking from the acceptance of some adverse outcomes as an inevitable result of delivered care to the concept of significant reduction or even elimination of such adverse outcomes [62]. The theory of care bundles is very close to the cycle of Deming Cycle of Change Plan, Do, Check, Act (PDCA) where there is repeated practice as well as careful monitoring for staff compliance with the care bundle and also the patient outcome to assess the effectiveness. Therefore, Care Bundles are frequently introduced to clinical practices as components of quality improvement initiatives [62].

15.2 Types of bundles

Care bundles are widely used in clinical practice to manage and prevent certain health conditions. **Table 6** shows the most common types of bundles and the areas where they can be applied:

15.3 Impact of using care bundles on clinical practice

Care bundles are one of the quality improvement initiatives that enhance the reliability of the care process which resulted in clinical outcomes improvement. They have great input on standardizing patient care processes and unifying clinical practice. In the infection prevention control field, bundles participated in reducing the negative outcomes that accompany the medical management process like hospital-acquired infections (HAIs). Antibiotic Care Bundle (ACB), for example, plays a significant role in implementing the antibiotic stewardship program that not only improves the proper use of antibiotics and optimizes the course of therapy, but also goes beyond to slowing the resistance of bacteria, decreasing the length of stay of patients and ultimately reducing the expenses of health care. Furthermore, each element of the bundle can be traced to assess the effectiveness of delivered care hence it provides reliable measures that can be used to see the areas required improvement.

15.4 Key points to implement successful care bundles

1. To improve effectiveness, bundles of care can be implemented in several phases: development or adoption, piloting, training, education, auditing, and feedback.

2. Collected data is used to assess the compliance of the staff or to see how bundles are effective and should be accessed, have a reliable collection

#	Care bundle	Where do they apply?
1	WHO Surgical Safety Checklists	Surgical theaters
2	Ventilator-Associated Pneumonia (VAP)	Intensive care units (ICU's)
3	Catheter-Associated Urinary Tract Infection (CAU-TI)	ICUs
4	A central line bloodstream infection (CLABSI)	ICUs
5	Peripheral Vascular Catheter (PVC)	All clinical area
6	Antibiotic Care Bundle (ACB-Bundle)	ICU's
7	Pressure Ulcer Prevention Care Bundle:	All areas of care where a patient is at risk for pressure ulcers.
8	Surgical Site Infection Prevention Bundle	ICUs, Surgical departments, isolation wards, etc.
9	Sepsis Care Bundle	ICUs, Isolation Wards, and all other areas where patients is vulnerable to sepsis.

Table 6.
Types of care bundles.

measure, validated, and analyzed in due course of time to guide the decision-making process.

3. Measurement should be accurate, consistent, and ongoing to authentically reflect hospital practice and, feedback should be delivered frequently (weekly or monthly if possible) to encourage improvement and sustainability [61].

4. To implement the bundle successfully, each element of the bundle must be implemented collectively with complete consistency to achieve the most favorable outcomes ("all or none" approach) [61].

5. Elements of the care bundle must be concise, simple, and prescriptive and neither static nor complex and hinder a successful adoption and implementation [63].

6. All of the elements of the bundle must be performed in a sequence by one healthcare team and within the same time frame.

7. Education, reminders audits, and feedback are the key components for the implementation of care bundles [64].

8. A flowchart is one of the useful quality tools that can be used to design care bundles [65].

9. Leadership support and staff commitment are the main success drivers of any care bundle.

16. Conclusion

Variations in healthcare are wide-ranging and can include an array of different treatment options, diagnostic procedures, and medication dosages that could jeopardize patient safety. Standardization can reduce variation and minimize the tendency of process failure. It also can enable shared learning, facilitate multi-disciplinary teamwork, and improve efficiency in interactions by establishing optimum conditions. Therefore, it is necessary to standardize healthcare processes, reducing variations in practice and minimizing the potential for risk or harm, this can be achieved by ongoing training, regular audits, and continuous improvement efforts, using care bundles, implementing standards of care, and following practice guidelines, policies, and procedures. And finally, having a dedicated quality culture to implement these initiatives, and achieve and sustain the desired improvement for the processes and system is the bedrock of this journey.

Acknowledgements

We thank Allah Almighty who gives me guidance and assistance to complete this work.

To all our families.

To everyone share their scientific insights and invaluable experiences in the healthcare improvement field.

To our colleagues whom we worked with and enriched our experiences.
And to all those who complete us...without them we are incomplete.

Conflict of interest

We hereby certify that there is not any actual or potential conflict of interest or unfair advantage at this time, in us providing the offer submission or performing the services required.

Thanks

We want to express our gratitude to all Intechopen team for their tireless efforts to guide and help us accomplish this work.

Acronyms and abbreviations

ACB	Antibiotic Care Bundle
A&E	accident & emergency
AI	artificial intelligence
CAU-TI	catheter associated urinary tract infection
CDC	communicable disease control
CIPP	Context, Input, Process, Product
CLABSI	Central Line-Associated Blood Stream Infection
CPGs	clinical practice guidelines
CQI	continuous quality improvement
EBM	evidence-based medicine
EI	emotional intelligence
ES	experiential style
FMEA	failure mode and effect analysis
GPSC	Global Patient Safety Collaborative
HAIs	hospital acquired infections
ICUs	intensive care units
ICPs	integrated care pathways
IHI	Institute of Healthcare Improvement
IOM	Institute of Medicine
ISQua	International Society for Quality in Healthcare
JCI	Joint Commission International
KPIs	Key Performance Indicators
NICE	National Institute for Health and Clinical Excellence
PDCA	Plan Do Check Act
PDSA	Plan Do Study Act
PPET	Patient, Provider, Environment, Task
P&Ps	policies & procedures
PVC	peripheral vascular catheter
QI	quality improvement
QMS	quality management system
RCA	Root Cause Analysis

RS	rational style
SOPs	Standardized Operating Protocols
STEEEP	Safe, Timely, Effective, Efficient, Equitable, Patient Centered
VAP	ventilated-associated pneumonia
WHO	World Health Organization
5S	Sort, Set, Shine, Standardize, Sustain

Author details

Mohammed M. Albaadani[1*], Adel Omar Bataweel[2], Alaa Mahmoud Ismail[3], Jameelah Mohammed Yaqoob[4], Ebrahim Sarwi Asiri[3], Hesham Ahmed Eid[5], Khaled M. Kasasbeh[3], Mohamed Fathy Shaban[6], Nasr Ali Mohammed[4], Samir Mohammed Bawazir[3], Siham Mohammed Saleh[7] and Yasser Sami Amer[8]

1 Health Watch Wigan and Leigh, United Kingdom

2 King Fahad Medical City, Riyadh, Saudi Arabia

3 Prince Sultan Military Medical City, Riyadh, Saudi Arabia

4 Ministry of Health and Population, Sana, Yemen

5 Founder of Quality Education Club, Cairo, Egypt

6 King Khaled Eye Specialist Hospital, Riyadh, Saudi Arabia

7 Prince Sultan Cardiac Center, Riyadh, Saudi Arabia

8 King Saud University Medical City, Riyadh, Saudi Arabia

*Address all correspondence to: albaadanim2@hotmail.com

IntechOpen

© 2024 The Author(s). Licensee IntechOpen. This chapter is distributed under the terms of the Creative Commons Attribution License (http://creativecommons.org/licenses/by/3.0), which permits unrestricted use, distribution, and reproduction in any medium, provided the original work is properly cited.

References

[1] To Err is Human. World Health Organization. 2012. p. 3. Available from: https://cdn.who.int/media/docs/default-source/patient-safety/curriculum-guide/resources/ps-curr-handouts/course03_handout_systems-and-the-effect-of-complexity-on-patient-care.pdf

[2] The NHS Patient Safety Strategy Safer Culture, Safer Systems, Safer Patients NHS England and NHS Improvement. NHS England; 2019. p. 84. Available from: https://www.england.nhs.uk/wp-content/uploads/2020/08/190708_Patient_Safety_Strategy_for_website_v4.pdf [Accessed: December 31, 2023]

[3] Understanding Importance of Quality Improvement in Healthcare. Enter. 2023. Available from: https://www.enter.health/post/understanding-importance-of-quality-improvement-in-healthcare [Accessed: December 5, 2023]

[4] Jabbal J. Embedding a culture of quality improvement. 2017. Available from: https://archive.kingsfund.org.uk/concern/published_works/000127887?locale=en [Accessed: December 5, 2023]

[5] Harold S. What is quality improvement in healthcare?. 2023. Available from: https://nursesgroup.co.uk/quality-improvement-in-healthcare [Accessed: December 5, 2023]

[6] Gupta BOV. Continuous Quality Improvement. 2023. Available from: https://www.ncbi.nlm.nih.gov/books/NBK559239/[Accessed: December 5, 2023]

[7] Hill JE, Stephani AM, Sapple P, Clegg AJ. The effectiveness of continuous quality improvement for developing professional practice and improving health care outcomes: A systematic review. Implementation Science. 2020;**15**(1):1-14. DOI: 10.1186/s13012-020-0975-2

[8] Continuous Improvement Explained | Wrike. Wrike. 2023. Available from: https://www.wrike.com/blog/explanation-continuous-improvement-examples/[Accessed: December 5, 2023]

[9] A Guide to Quality Improvement Tools [Internet]. London: Healthcare Quality Improvement Partnership Ltd. (HQIP); 2020. Available from: https://www.hqip.org.uk/wp-content/uploads/2021/01/Final-Quality-Improvement-QI-Tools-09-12-20.pdf [Accessed: December 31, 2023]

[10] Healthcare variation | Australian Commission on Safety and Quality in Health Care. Australian Commission on Safety and Quality in Health Care. 2023. Available from: https://www.safetyandquality.gov.au/our-work/healthcare-variation [Accessed: December 31, 2023]

[11] Reducing Clinical Variation. EvidenceCare. 2023. Available from: https://evidence.care/clinical-variation/ [Accessed: December 31, 2023]

[12] Reduce Variability of Care: Factors, Benefits and Methods [Internet]. Baltimore, Maryland, USA: Wolters Kluwer. 13 Mar 2019;1. Available from: https://www.wolterskluwer.com/en/expert-insights/reduce-variability-of-care-factors-benefits-and-methods [Accessed: December 31, 2023]

[13] Djulbegovic B, Guyatt GH. Progress in evidence-based medicine: A quarter century on. The Lancet. 2017;**390**(10092):415-423

[14] Lavelle J, Schast A, Keren R. Standardizing care processes and improving quality using pathways and continuous quality improvement. Current Treatment Options in Pediatrics. 2015;**1**(4):347-358. DOI: 10.1007/s40746-015-0026-4

[15] Peters S, Sukumar K, Blanchard S, Ramasamy A, Malinowski J, Ginex P, et al. Trends in guideline implementation: An updated scoping review. Implementation Science. 2022;**17**(1):50

[16] Glasziou P, Ogrinc G, Goodman S. Can evidence-based medicine and clinical quality improvement learn from each other? BMJ Quality and Safety. 2011;**20**(Suppl 1):i13-i17

[17] El Mikati IK, Khabsa J, Harb T, Khamis M, Agarwal A, Pardo-Hernandez H, et al. A framework for the development of living practice guidelines in health care. Annals of Internal Medicine. 2022;**175**(8):1154-1160

[18] Correa VC, Lugo-Agudelo LH, Aguirre-Acevedo DC, Contreras JAP, Borrero AMP, Patiño-Lugo DF, et al. Individual, health system, and contextual barriers and facilitators for the implementation of clinical practice guidelines: A systematic metareview. Health Research Policy and Systems. 2020;**18**(1):1-11. DOI: 10.1186/s12961-020-00588-8

[19] Beauchemin M, Cohn E, Shelton RC. Implementation of clinical practice guidelines in the health care setting: A concept analysis. ANS. Advances in Nursing Science. 2019;**42**(4):307-324. Available from: https://pubmed.ncbi.nlm.nih.gov/30839334/

[20] Joint Commission International. Joint Commission on Accreditation of Healthcare Organizations. Joint Commission International Accreditation Standards for Hospitals. 7th ed. Illinoi: Joint Commission Resources; 2020. pp. 1-391

[21] Consultancy Improvement Support, Policies and Procedures Review. Social Care Institute for Excellence. 2024. Available from: https://www.scie.org.uk/consultancy/policies-procedures-review [Accessed: January 1, 2024]

[22] Importance of Hospital Policies and Procedures | PowerDMS. powerdms. 2020. Available from: https://www.powerdms.com/policy-learning-center/importance-of-policies-and-procedures-for-hospitals [Accessed: January 1, 2024]

[23] Top 5 Types of Healthcare Policies and Procedures. RLDatix. 2020. Available from: https://resources.rldatix.com/en-us-blog/types-of-hospital-policies-and-procedures [Accessed: January 1, 2024]

[24] Shaw SLF. Leadership for Change. 2nd ed. Geneva: International Council of Nurses; 2007. pp. 1-112

[25] Gattnar E, Ekinci O, Detschew V. Clinical process modeling and performance measurement in hospitals. In: 2011 IEEE 15th International Enterprise Distributed Object Computing Conference Workshops [Internet]. Helsinki, Finland: IEEE; 2011. pp. 132-140. Available from: http://ieeexplore.ieee.org/document/6037612/

[26] Melissa Welch KM. Standardizing Excellence: Top 5 Pillars to Reduce Unwarranted Care Variation. Health Catalyst. 2024. Available from: https://www.healthcatalyst.com/insights/standardizing-excellence-five-pillars-reducing-unwarranted-care-variation [Accessed: January 1, 2024]

[27] Guidance on Developing Key Performance Indicators and Minimum

Data Sets to Monitor Healthcare Quality [Internet]. Dublin: Health Information and Quality Authority; 2013. Available from: https://www.hiqa.ie/sites/default/files/2017-01/KPI-Guidance-Version1.1-2013.pdf [Accessed: January 1, 2024]

[28] Manaher S. Benchmark vs Standard: Deciding Between Similar Terms. The Content Authority. 2024. Available from: https://thecontentauthority.com/blog/benchmark-vs-standard [Accessed: January 1, 2024]

[29] Reducing Clinical Variation | Healthcare Challenges | Wolters Kluwer. Wolters Kluwer. 2024. Available from: https://www.wolterskluwer.com/en-gb/know/healthcare-challenges/reducing-clinical-variation [Accessed: January 1, 2024]

[30] Improvement Coach Professional Development Program [Internet]. Boston, USA: Institute for Healthcare Improvement (IHI); 2023. pp. 1-87. Available from: https://www.ihi.org/education/InPersonTraining/ImprovementCoach/Improvement-Coach/Pages/default.aspx

[31] The 5S method - Optimising the workplace | IAPM. International Association of Project Managers (IAPM). 2024. Available from: https://www.iapm.net/en/blog/5s-method/ [Accessed: January 1, 2024]

[32] Islam S, Islam Q, Rahman A, Huq A, Hassan A, Yoshimura Y, et al. Manual for Implementation of 5S in Hospital Setting [Internet]. Dhaka: TQM Unit, Hospital Services Management, DGHS; 2015. p. 12. Available from: www.hsmdghs-bd.org [Accessed: January 1, 2024]

[33] Miller D. Patient safety lessons from LEAN manufacturing | Fierce Healthcare. fiercehealthcare. 2013. Available from: https://www.fiercehealthcare.com/hospitals/patient-safety-lessons-from-lean-manufacturing [Accessed: January 1, 2024]

[34] Kanamori S, Shibanuma A, Jimba M. Applicability of the 5S management method for quality improvement in health-care facilities: A review. Trop. Medicine & Health. 2016;**44**(1):21. DOI: 10.1186/s41182-016-0022-9

[35] Shahali S, Khajehasani M, Torabipoor A, Ahmadiangali K. The impact of applying 5S management method on patient satisfaction in healthcare centers' services. Research Square [Internet]. 2019;**8**(4):197-202. DOI: 10.21203/rs.2.14598/v1 [Accessed: January 1, 2024]

[36] Kanamori S, Sow S, Castro MC, Matsuno R, Tsuru A, Jimba M. Implementation of 5S management method for lean healthcare at a health center in Senegal: A qualitative study of staff perception. Global Health Action. 2015;**8**(1):27256. DOI: 10.3402/gha.v8.27256

[37] 5S in Healthcare. Redesigning Care. 2013. Available from: www.flinders.sa.gov.au/redesigningcare [Accessed: January 8, 2024]

[38] Leotsakos A, Zheng H, Croteau R, Loeb JM, Sherman H, Hoffman C, et al. Standardization in patient safety: The WHO high 5s project. International Journal for Quality in Health Care. 2014;**26**(2):109-116. DOI: 10.1093/intqhc/mzu010

[39] Patient Safety. World Health Organization. 2023. Available from: https://www.who.int/news-room/fact-sheets/detail/patient-safety [Accessed: January 1, 2024]

[40] Tingle J. Global patient safety initiatives and the NHS. British Journal of

Nursing [Internet]. 2020;**29**(11). Available from: https://www.britishjournalofnursing.com/content/patient-safety/global-patient-safety-initiatives-and-the-nhs [Accessed: January 1, 2024]

[41] High 5s: Action on Patient Safety. World Health Organization. 2024;1. Available from: https://www.high5s.org/bin/view/Main/WebHome [Accessed: January 1, 2024]

[42] World Health Organization (WHO). The High 5s Project Interim Report [Internet]. Geneva: World Health Organization; 2014. Available from: https://iris.who.int/bitstream/handle/10665/330068/9789241507257-eng.pdf?sequence=1 [Accessed: January 1, 2024]

[43] Esposito P, Canton AD. Clinical audit, a valuable tool to improve quality of care: General methodology and applications in nephrology. World. Journal of Nephrology. 2014;**3**(4):249

[44] Clinical Audit Definition & Cycle [Internet]. Radar Healthcare. 2022. Available from: https://radarhealthcare.com/news-blogs/clinical-audit-definition-and-cycle/ [Accessed: January 3, 2024]

[45] Conducting a Clinical Audit. The Royal College of Pathologists. 2024. Available from: https://www.rcpath.org/profession/patient-safety-and-quality-improvement/conducting-a-clinical-audit.html [Accessed: January 1, 2024]

[46] Limb C, Fowler A, Gundogan B, Koshy K, Agha R. How to conduct a clinical audit and quality improvement project. International Journal of Surgical Oncology (NY). 2017;**2**(6):e24. Available from: https://journals.lww.com/ijsoncology/fulltext/2017/07000/how_to_conduct_a_clinical_audit_and_quality.5.aspx [Accessed: January 1, 2024]

[47] Bataweel AO, Bataweel AO. The impact of medical profession type, gender, and years of experience on thinking styles: What are the implications for patient safety? Journal of Behavioral and Brain Science. 2022;**12**(11):569-588. Available from: http://www.scirp.org/journal/PaperInformation.aspx?PaperID=121122 [Accessed: January 1, 2024]

[48] Bataweel AO, Ahmed MGM, Bataweel AO, Ahmed MGM. Exploring emotional intelligence and thinking style in Saudi residents: A cross-sectional study. Psychology. 2023;**14**(2):158-180. Available from: http://www.scirp.org/journal/PaperInformation.aspx?PaperID=123033 [Accessed: January 1, 2024]

[49] Bataweel AO. Personality traits, thinking styles, and emotional intelligence in nursing, towards healthcare providers' characterization and safer patient care. Open Nursing Journal. 2023;**13**(02):130-166. DOI: 10.4236/ojn.2023.132009

[50] Bataweel AO, BinOthaimeen N. Personality traits, thinking style, and emotional intelligence among pharmacy staff towards safer patient care. Psychology. 2023;**14**(06):1015-1032. DOI: 10.4236/psych.2023.146054

[51] Bataweel AO, Al GK, Al AF, Bataweel AO, Al GK, Al AF. Counterproductive work Behaviors in a Saudi tertiary healthcare organization. Psychology. 2023;**14**(12):1768-1792. Available from: http://www.scirp.org/journal/PaperInformation.aspx?PaperID=129729 [Accessed: January 9, 2024]

[52] Ben-Zion Z, Korem N, Spiller TR, Duek O, Keynan JN, Admon R, et al. Longitudinal volumetric evaluation of hippocampus and amygdala subregions

in recent trauma survivors. Molecular Psychiatry. 2022;**28**(2):657-667. Available from: https://www.nature.com/articles/s41380-022-01842-x [Accessed: January 1, 2024]

[53] Phillips RD, De Bellis MD, Brumback T, Clausen AN, Clarke-Rubright EK, Haswell CC, et al. Volumetric trajectories of hippocampal subfields and amygdala nuclei influenced by adolescent alcohol use and lifetime trauma. Translational Psychiatry. 2021;**11**(1):1-13. Available from: https://www.nature.com/articles/s41398-021-01275-0 [Accessed: January 1, 2024]

[54] Schwabe L. Memory under stress: From single systems to network changes. European Journal of Neuroscience. 2017;**45**(4):478-489. DOI: 10.1111/ejn.13478

[55] Taylor J. Importance of Staff Training in Health and Social Care. The Access Group. 2023. Available from: https://www.theaccessgroup.com/en-gb/blog/hsc-importance-of-staff-training-in-health-and-social-care/ [Accessed: January 1, 2024]

[56] Evidence scan: Quality improvement training for healthcare professionals. 2012. Available from: https://www.health.org.uk/sites/default/files/QualityImprovementTrainingForHealthcareProfessionals.pdf [Accessed: January 1, 2024]

[57] Improving Safety Through Education and Training. 2016. Available from: www.hee.nhs.uk/the-commission-on-education-and-training-for-patient-safety [Accessed: January 1, 2024]

[58] Evaluation of Training. 2024. Available from: https://pib.gov.in/PressReleseDetailm.aspx?PRID=1763318 [Accessed: January 1, 2024]

[59] Shaw CD. Accreditation Definitions | EBMT. The International Society for Quality in Health Care. 2004. Available from: https://www.ebmt.org/accreditation-definitions [Accessed: January 1, 2024]

[60] Standards for JCI Accreditation | Joint Commission International. The Joint Commission International. Available from: https://www.jointcommissioninternational.org/standards [Accessed: January 1, 2024]

[61] Sean Wasserman AM. Guide to Infection Control in the Healthcare Setting Bundles in Infection Prevention and Safety. Gonzalo Bearman, editor. International Society for Infectious Diseases; 2018. 1-15 p. Available from: https://isid.org/guide/infectionprevention/bundles/ [Accessed: January 1, 2024]

[62] Clarkson DMG. The role of 'care bundles' in healthcare. British Journal of Healthcare Management. 2013;**19**(2):63-68. DOI: 10.12968/bjhc.2013.19.2.63

[63] Chehab Hussein D. Bundles of Care. Dubai: Dubai Hospital; 2019. pp. 1-36

[64] Borgert MJ, Goossens A, Dongelmans DA. What are effective strategies for the implementation of care bundles on ICUs: A systematic review. Implementation Science. 2015;**10**(1):119. DOI: 10.1186/s13012-015-0306-1

[65] Borgert M, Binnekade J, Paulus F, Goossens A, Dongelmans D. A flowchart for building evidence-based care bundles in intensive care: Based on a systematic review. International Journal for Quality in Health Care. 2017;**29**(2):163-175. DOI: 10.1093/intqhc/mzx009

Chapter 7

Long Wait Times at Hospitals in Jamaica: A Potential Risk to Patient Safety

Opal Davidson, James Fallah, Denice Curtis and Chukwuma Richard Uzoka

Abstract

Long wait time in public emergency rooms continues to be a major challenge in the Jamaican healthcare system. The aim of the study is to investigate the risk management strategies implemented by other nations in maintaining patient safety. The research method is a descriptive analytic study using literature review design to examine current and historical data to identify solutions to the long wait time at hospitals in Jamaica. The results revealed that adequate use and evaluation of risk management strategies, continuous upgrading of national emergency care health policy, improving triage systems, decreasing overcrowding and proper use of observation units in the ER, and maximizing the use of current technology to improve patient care do decrease the threat to patient safety. In conclusion, implementation of the risk management approach developed in this study can assist in maintaining patient safety by decreasing long wait time in public hospitals across the globe.

Keywords: long wait time, Jamaica public hospitals, emergency care, patient safety, risk management strategies

1. Introduction

Waiting time can be defined as the period covering the arrival of the patient to the emergency department until when the patient is provided with the required treatment by a qualified medical professional. On an average the wait time for all emergency room departments in the world is four hours [1]. Long wait times in emergency rooms at public hospitals can significantly impact patient health [2]. Similarly, decreasing the waiting time at accident and emergency (A & E) departments for patients utilizing health care services at public hospitals in Jamaica is a major challenge. Despite this fact, one of the national strategic policy priorities of the Ministry of Health & Wellness (MOHW) in Jamaica is to provide quality assurance in the delivery of health services to the population. Hence, the importance of satisfactorily addressing the challenge of long wait time in public hospitals in Jamaica. However, there are several factors that do contribute to this reality of long wait time that include (1) overcrowding of patients in the emergency room may result in increased workload

IntechOpen

on staff coverage [3], (2) insufficient space and accommodation for patients, (3) shortage in beds in the emergency room, (4) insufficient labour force, (5) poor time management by medical team, (6) absenteeism of the labour force, (7) inadequate triage procedures, along with poor patient medical records management and lack of electronic medical records [4]. Additionally, the MOHW has implemented new measures that include training, installation of electronic medical recording system, and improvement in equipment and spacing to address the ongoing problem of overcrowding in the hospitals. Thus, there is the need for the ministry of health to further prioritize financial investment in the public health sector in Jamaica.

Hence, the aim of this study is to further investigate this phenomenon of long wait time in the public hospitals in Jamaica that threatens the quality of health care delivery and management. Also, from completion of the study it is intended that further recommendations will be made, on how the long wait time at public hospitals in Jamaica can be decreased or be eliminated over time. Additionally, in seeking to investigate the unfortunate phenomenon of long wait hours in the Jamaican public hospitals, risk management strategies will be identified to aid in minimizing or preventing potential risks to patient safety.

Also, it is anticipated that the findings obtained from this study when shared will be beneficial in emergency care management across the world through the World Health Organization (WHO).

2. Methodology

The research method for this study is a descriptive analytic study using literature review design exploring databases such as Google Scholar, reputable international journals such as Science Direct, Proquest, Pubmed, EBSCO, BMJ Open and others. Key words or themes were explored to gather the data using secondary data online that included: Risk factors to Patient safety, Long Wait Time, Jamaica Hospitals, Triage, Healthcare Management and Supervision, risk management strategies, patient safety, and accident and emergency departments in Jamaica and other countries were used to source the required information using the various online databases. The selection criteria for articles: mainly peer reviewed articles were referenced. Also, credible newspaper publications were included to support the information provided that could not be sourced elsewhere.

3. Background to the problem

The various challenges facing the Jamaican health care system over many years, cannot be overlooked. These major problems include growing long wait periods in patients receiving the required treatment at many of the public hospitals across the health sector in Jamaica [5].

More so, with the gradual introduction of the concept of universal coverage in the health care system of Jamaica through two main policy interventions by Ministry of Health & Wellness in Jamaica (MOHW), namely the National Health Fund (NHF) in 2003 and the removal of user fees in accessing health care services in 2008, the existing problem of long wait time has been further compounded. As a result of the implementation of these much needed interventions more Jamaicans have been accessing the health care services at the various public hospitals across the country. According to Dr. Coombs, a leading public health doctor in Western Regional Health Authority (WRHA), there has been a steady increase in the health care services offered to the general public over the past 10 years that include diagnostic services by 314% and pharmacy by 71%. With such major development in the health care sector, more individuals over time would inevitably seek medical assistance with the significant improvement seen in the health care delivery system in Jamaica over the years [6].

Recently, a reporter for the Jamaica Gleaner commented that the hospital managers must be blamed for the long wait time due to unsatisfactory organizational management of human and other resources in managing the health care services offered to patients. However, St. Andrade Sinclairs, the acting regional director of the Western Regional Health Authorities (WRHA) disagreed since he believes that "such generalization is impractical and does not apply in all cases" [7]. However, Dr. Taleya Girvan, a Pediatrician who works in the A & E department at the Bustamante Hospital for Children (BHC), contended that the long wait time for patients in A & E departments is not unique to Jamaica but it is a common phenomenon across the world. In her view, the long wait time is the result of the triage process. The less urgent the case, the waiting time will be longer. Another confounding problem identified by Dr. Girvan is the acceptance in the A & E department for all categories of illness, which further complicates the existing problem in long wait time, since patients that can be seen by their private practitioners or at the health centers are receiving treatment in the A & E departments. These patients should otherwise be seen at their health centers or be asked to attend a specialized clinic [8]. Evidently, the problem of long wait time in A & E departments in Jamaica is complex and multifaceted, so there is no one-fix solution. Hence, the importance of this study that will seek to further investigate the existing challenges the health care system faces at the present moment and to identify strategies and solutions for improving the patient-provider encounter issue.

4. Areas covered in the study

4.1 Ensuring patient safety

The WHO defined patient safety as 'the absence of preventable harm to a patient during the process of health care' [9, 10]. According to Ackroyd-Stolarz et al., there is a distinctive association between the length of wait time in the emergency room and the risk of hospital admission or death in the elderly patients [11, 12]. Thus, the importance of ensuring patient safety in hospitals in Jamaica since overcrowding in the A & E departments remains a major challenge. More so, patients have always been complaining about long wait time in hospitals across Jamaica and still such complaints have not resulted in any significant improvements in the health care system [12]. In fact, the MOHW in Jamaica has recently informed all Jamaicans to brace themselves for longer waiting time for the end of the year and going forward into 2024 [13]. Such news are not welcoming nor encouraging and so promoting the implementation of key strategies to decrease the waiting time in Jamaican public hospitals must be pursued and encouraged.

4.2 Effects of long wait time in A & E

A disorganized triage system is a major contributing factor to the long wait time of an average of over 4 hours in the emergency rooms on a global scale. Patients are often dissatisfied with the triage process and the medical teams are often disheartened by the outcome themselves [13, 14]. Also, Nyce et al., postulates that prolonged wait times are associated with worse patient experience with discharged patients from emergency departments [12, 15].

4.3 Risk management strategies

Risk management strategies in the Jamaican public hospital emergency rooms are essential in ensuring patient safety, since it requires implementing key guidelines to safeguard and alert health care providers in making needed changes, to provide the highest quality medical and nursing care in preventing patient injuries. Similarly, such strategies are crucial when caring for patients in an emergency care setting. Important to the risk management process are five common strategies for managing risk which are avoidance, retention, transferring, sharing, and loss reduction. Each technique aims to address and reduce risk while understanding that risk is impossible to eliminate completely [16]. Hence, the investigation of the long wait time in hospitals in Jamaica, should assist in identifying these key risk management strategies that should be used to improve the quality of care and patient safety on a global scale.

5. Original theoretical framework of risk management for A & E

As a result of the absence of a universal theoretical approach to the management of risk factors and patient safety in A & E departments on a global scale, an original theoretical framework has been developed for the purpose of this study. The concept of risk management is not new and has been used globally in the world of business with much success. Applying it to the field of health care should not be a major challenge. Therefore, it is anticipated that this model will be adopted globally, to further improve the quality of health care delivery and management. This health care delivery model will aid in the early detection and addressing of any key risk factors that may be contributing to long wait time in the emergency room setting that may negatively impact patient safety. Risk management can be defined as the process of analyzing processes and practices that are in place, identifying risk factors, and implementing procedures to address those risks [17]. More so, the World Health Organization in 2019 has approved a global patient safety action plan covering the period 2021–2030. The aim is to ensure that all health care systems are on board in promoting patient safety in health care that includes emergency care for all nations [18]. **Figure 1** illustrates the risk management and patient safety model developed for A & E departments worldwide.

5.1 Utilization of the conceptual framework

5.1.1 Assessment of risk factors

The process of assessment of risk factors impacting long wait time in A & E departments does require the coordinated effort of all members of the health team, even though it is primarily the responsibility of supervisory management. Especially, since these risk factors are many and they may occur at varying times during a work shift in the emergency room. These risk factors include (1) overcrowding may results in the increase in workload that affects staff coverage, (2) insufficient space and accommodation for patients, (3) shortage in beds, (4) insufficient labour force,

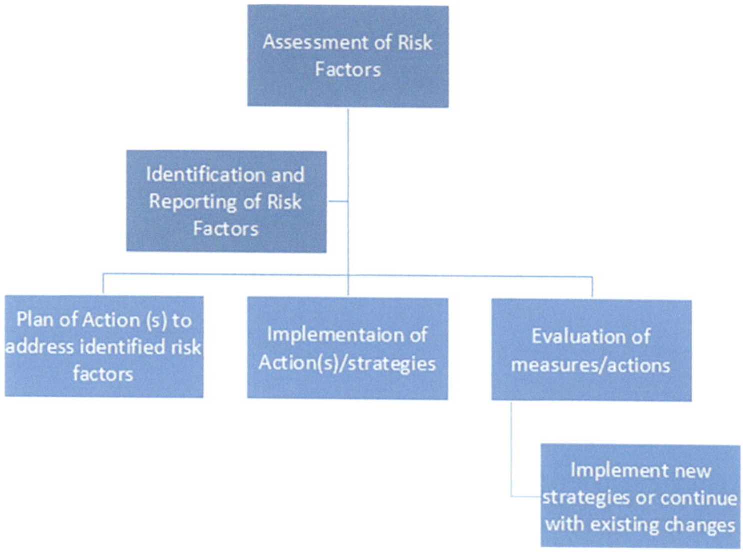

Figure 1.
Risk management strategies and patient safety management framework: an A & E perspective developed by Dr. Opal Davidson 27.11.2023.

(5) poor time management by medical team, (6) absenteeism of the labour force and (7) inadequate triage procedures. Early identification of these risk factors and implementation of the appropriate interventions in time to avert any major health care challenges is ultimately the ideal solution to decreasing the long wait time in hospitals [19]. However, as health care providers it is difficult to achieve this feat. Still every effort should be made to do all that is possible to safeguard the quality of health care that is provided to all patients in ensuring their safety.

5.1.2 Identification and reporting of risk factors

It is highly recommended that an established system for identifying risk factors be established in the A & E departments. A variety of formats do exist that may involve the use of technology, or a charting system using a whiteboard and other forms of documentation. Also, there must be an established protocol for reporting these identified risk factors so that the required solutions can be provided, allowing for enhanced problem-solving to occur from all levels of the health care system. This means that there must be open and efficient communication throughout the health sector. Below is a diagram that illustrates the open communication and collaboration that should exist among the various levels of the health care sector, to address the challenge for example of shortage of beds in A & E department, using Falmouth hospital in WRHA for the illustration in **Figure 2**.

It is important that this form of health care organized communication and collaboration include the entire health care sector, thereby, allowing the A & E departments to receive the necessary assistance in advance such as equipment, beds, and labour force to prevent major challenges in providing efficient patient care and decreasing long wait time. Also, there must be effective communication from the point of the A & E departments in Jamaica internally at public hospitals and with the wider health care sector. Effective communication means the relaying of information in regards to the need of

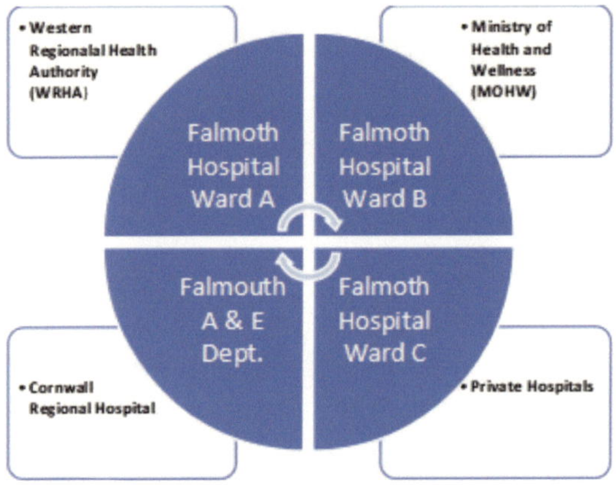

Figure 2.
Illustrates an example of the open communication and collaboration that should exist between A & E departments from the level of the wards at hospitals to the wider health care sector in addressing the existing risk factors. Developed by Dr. O. Davidson 19.12.2023.

the A & E department for example as shown in **Figure 2** with the ministry of health and the private health sector. Thereby allowing the A& E departments to be linked with the required staff and equipment to ensure that health care staff, medical procedures and equipment are available to decrease the wait time for patients. Patients can also be referred to other health care facilities for further management of their health conditions.

5.1.3 Plan of action to address identified risk factors

There must be clear guidelines of how interventions regarding specific risk factors must be handled since deviations may result in the creation of unseen problems. These guidelines must be tested, tried, and proven to work in the given A & E department, since no two settings are the same. Plan of action should be a team effort to ensure the involvement of all the team members since they will be empowered, having been a part of the planning process. It is important therefore, that each team member is committed to the success of the plans that have been developed to improve patient safety in the emergency care setting.

5.1.4 Implementation of interventions

Before implementation of the plan, it must be clearly stated who is responsible for completing a particular task, which will prevent unnecessary confusion and will enable greater accountability of team members. Implementation must be time bound and properly executed for improved outcome. Communication among team members is vital at this point. Ongoing observation, documentation and follow up is crucial at this time. The literature shows that there are already proven and established steps to complete when implementing a health care intervention to enhance patient safety in Jamaican emergency rooms [20].

5.1.5 Evaluation of interventions

In order to evaluate, clear goals would have to be set in regards to the problem being addressed and an outline of the desired outcomes would have to be established.

Supervisory management is responsible for this aspect, but all medical team members should be engaged in the process. Accurate determination of the outcome of health care interventions allows the healthcare team the opportunity to become more knowledgeable in order to improve the services being offered and to inform future healthcare policy making and the implementation of new protocols to maintain patient safety. Data collection is the process that is used to guide the evaluation process using various research methods, appropriate for the study. Data gathering can be obtained from varying sources that include patients' records, direct feedback from patients, observation, and other forms of documentation [21].

5.1.6 Implementation of new interventions

On evaluation, if the desired outcome was not achieved from the intervention implemented for decreasing waiting times in the Jamaican emergency care and patient safety. It is important that reassessment of the risk factors be conducted to ensure that the medical needs of the patients are met. Therefore, a new plan of action must be considered and be implemented. If the evaluation is being achieved but more interventions are needed to achieve the desired outcome, then they should be implemented as well.

6. Result and discussion

6.1 Comparative waiting times in other countries including emergency care

It is essential to note that the long waiting time for patients to receive treatment in the accident and emergency department is not unique to Jamaica but is of growing concern for health care delivery on a global scale. It is important to reveal that there are three countries mentioned by the Organization for Economic Cooperation and Development (OECD) as having the shortest wait times for patients receiving health care and they are notably Switzerland, Netherlands, and Germany, with 88%, 87%, and 87% of patients, respectively, generally being seen in 1 day or less, as shown in **Figure 3.**

6.1.1 Germany

This country spends very large resources on providing accessible health care for its citizens. However, the quality of healthcare is only average based on the OECD findings, thus impacting waiting times and emergency care. Since there is a gradual decline in public health care with private health care slowly taking over [20, 23]. In comparison in Jamaica the public hospitals remain the main emergency care for its citizens.

6.1.2 Switzerland

This country has a small but growing private health sector, since the health care system is primarily publicly owned. Expenditure in healthcare is high and its infrastructure is highly modernized with the installation of digitization, electronic health records, health information exchange system and telemedicine. The focus is more on ambulatory care and there is a decrease in the length of inpatient stay. Centralization

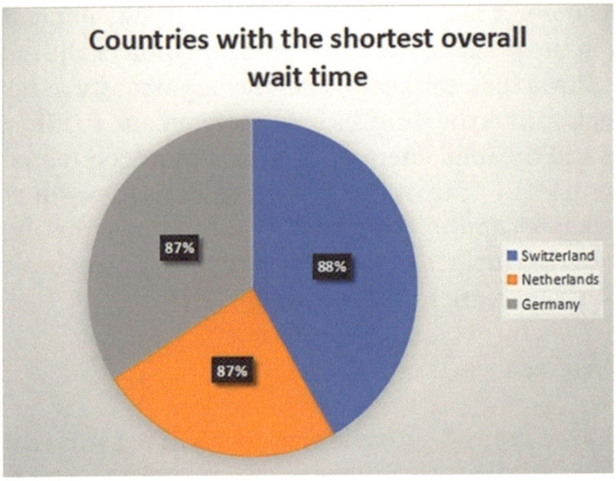

Figure 3.
The top 3 ranked countries with the shortest overall wait time providing health care reported by OECD in 2023 [22].

of the pharmaceutical system is the focus. Challenges exist in digitization and data management due to financial constraints and labor shortage [20, 23]. Similarly, in Jamaica the private sector emergency care is not as developed and therefore the citizens rely primarily on the emergency care provided by the public hospitals.

6.1.3 The Netherlands

The Dutch government provides universal health insurance system that has a public and private insurance component. The government has modernized their health care system which is paying off. Highly modernized technology and first-class treatment exist to attract patients and has significantly decreased the waiting times for healthcare with 87% of the individuals being seen by a medical provider in 1 day or less [20, 23]. However, the concept of universal coverage in the health care system in Jamaica since 2008, does not provide insurance coverage for its citizens. The cost of emergency care in Jamaica for citizens is covered by the government, however patients with health insurance are required to pay.

6.1.4 United Kingdom

The United Kingdom has experienced an existing health care problem of long wait time that affects the quality of health care delivery and management. Therefore, the National Health Service (NHS) has sought to make improvements in the waiting time by requiring that at least 95% of patients attending A & E be admitted, transferred, or discharged within 4 hours [24]. In December 2022, an intermediary threshold target of 76% to be hit by March 2024 was introduced with further improvement expected in 2024/25. The change evidently reflected the impact of COVID -19. It is worth noting that significant changes were being made to the protocol that guides the operations in the A & E since in March 2019, the Review of NHS Access Standards was published. The review proposed that the current four-hour A & E target should be replaced by a set of access standards, including the average waiting time in A & E, time to initial clinical assessment, and time to emergency treatment for critically ill and injured patients. The aim of the changes inevitably is to ensure better monitoring of the waiting time in the A & E departments. These changes were short-lived since, in September 2022, Thérèse Coffey, the Health Secretary repealed the change so that the existing four-hour target remains [25].

6.1.5 Canada

In Canada, Lakeridge Health's ED Wait Times Tracker was created to assist patients in getting quality health care in a shorter time span and to predict the estimated wait time to see a doctor in the ED. However, the tracker is unable to predict the length of stay since the patient may be required further tests and treatment which may increase the length of the visit [26].

6.1.6 United States of America

In the United States the average wait time in A & E departments is an hour and a half for the patient to be taken to their room and 2.25 hours before being discharged. Furthermore, the median time for receiving pain medication in the ED for patients with an extremity fracture is 72 minutes [27]. Moreover, the number of patients who leave the department without being seen has sharply increased in recent years, some of them being seriously ill. One of the reasons the patients have reported for leaving is the long waiting times in the ED (Mean = 6.4 hours) [28].

Some recommendations to fix the problem include (1) increasing the number of staff who conduct triage in the ED; (2) enabling transparency in information, (3) providing equitable workload and (4) utilizing a team-based care model [29]. More so, the implementation of quality improvement measures such as engaging the use of a data driven approach with support from senior clinicians and constant feedback on outcomes was highly recommended [30].

6.1.7 The Caribbean

Long wait time in the emergency departments in the Caribbean remains an important challenge as well. In Trinidad and Tobago in 2020 a qualitative study led by Freitas et al., investigated the flow of patients in an emergency department to identify the main contributing factors that were affecting patient turnover in that health care setting. The findings indicated organizational processes such as streaming, front loading of investigations and the transferring process of patients were major factors impacting the turnover time of patients in the emergency department [31]. The streaming process in the ED was first implemented in England to place patients into queues according to the level of acuity [32]. The study conducted by Freitas et al., used the Canadian Triage and Acuity Scale (CTAS) to allocate the patients to queues. The front load of investigations refers to the point of care tests (ECGs, urine tests, X-rays for minor injuries) that should be ordered during the triage process and before the patients are allocated into queues. This approach has resulted in decreased wait times and enhanced patient satisfaction and safety.

Correspondingly, in Barbados the challenge of long wait time continues to escalate. However, the country is making every effort to address the problem through transparency. Since as recent as November 2023, the newspaper Barbados Today highlighted that there is a public notice sent by the Ministry of Health announcing that the wait time at Queen Elizabeth Hospital emergency room will be increased. The notice clearly stated the category of patients that will be seen immediately as outlined by the triage system. These patients include cases such as accidents, sight threatening complaints, gunshot wounds, heart attacks, active seizures, or patients requiring resuscitation [33].

Further studies into the healthcare management of these nations in maintaining the shortest wait time in health care should be explored and the information be made available for other nations to benefit. In addition, the impact of national health policies regarding waiting time in hospitals should be explored.

7. Recommended solutions

7.1 The psychological effects of long wait time

An essential study was conducted by Lee & Yoon in November, 2023 suggests patients do experience high levels of anxiety while waiting for medical care in emergency rooms. The study purports that using nature to enhance the environment while patients wait assists in significantly decreasing the level of anxiety using plants, nature images and a combination of both interventions [34].

Studies have shown that patients with mental health illness experience longer waiting times (16.5–21.5 hours) than those without a mental health disease which shows the disparity of care for this particularly vulnerable group [35].

7.2 Recommended risk management strategies

It is a fact that health care services can also benefit from shorter wait times at hospitals, since patient turnover improves on the use of resources and is more cost effective [36]. More so, the patients generally leave the health care facility more satisfied and are, therefore, more likely to return. Patients will also be more willing to encourage others to use the health care service, thereby improving their quality of life and that of others [37]. In addition, the WHO reported that many OECD countries have taken measures to reduce waiting times in hospitals through additional funding but with mixed success [38].

Therefore, to improve the wait time, every country should make an effort to develop a national health policy that includes a platform for better management of their health care issues impacting emergency care and waiting time. A risk management approach is recommended to ensure the interventions are preventive rather than corrective in nature.

Next, the use of technology in creating a reporting and alert system for A & E departments within all countries is necessary. Thus, ensuring that the needs of these emergency departments can be addressed in a timely manner.

7.3 Decreasing the psychological impact of long wait time

During COVID-19 it was evident that mentally ill patients were in need of more psychological support while waiting for completion of specific procedures such as Magnetic Resonance Imaging (MRI). The main reasons presented were the high level of anxiety and the increased risk of injury to the patient. A research study conducted in 2021 revealed that patients felt that their psychological needs could have been addressed more through the following implementations: acknowledgement of their concerns, peer support, and periodic communication about wait-list position, prioritization criteria and anticipated procedure date [39]. Similarly, long wait times in emergency rooms that do negatively impact the psychological state of patients requires interventions to ease the adverse effects that include anxiety, depression, increased stress levels, morbidity and even death. According to Shen & Lee 2018 a team-based approach that involves closer communication and coordination between patients and the care provider will result in more positive patient outcomes [40].

7.4 Improving triage systems

Separating critical and non-critical patients in the waiting room can help, as low-acuity patients may be able to be treated in another area [41]. Triage is a process that is critical to the effective management of modern emergency departments. Triage systems aim not only to ensure that the patient receive the required emergency care, but also to provide an effective tool for departmental organization, monitoring, and evaluation [39]. Globally, over the last 20 years, triage systems have been standardized in a number of countries and efforts made to ensure consistency of application. It is also noted that the ongoing crowding of emergency departments resulting from access block and increased demand has led to calls for a review of systems of triage. In addition, international variance in triage systems limits the capacity for bench marking [42]. The basic premise of Triage is primarily the sorting of patients for treatment in situations of least modest resource scarcity, according to an assessment of the patient's medical condition and the application of an established sorting system or plan [43]. Defined in this way, the most common types of triage include emergency department triage, inpatient (ICU) triage, incident (multicausality) triage, military (battlefield) triage, and disaster (mass casualty) triage [44]. All the listed types of triage have distinctive elements such as: (1) modest scarcity of health care resources exists, (2) assesses each patient's medical needs, usually based on a brief examination and (3) the use of an established system or plan, usually based on an algorithm or a set of criteria, to determine a specific treatment or treatment priority for each patient by the health care provider [44, 45]. In 2016, the Ministry of Health and Wellness in Jamaica selected the Emergency Severity Index as the triage tool to be used nationally. The Emergency Severity Index (ESI) is a 5-level triage tool validated and used in more than 70% of emergency departments in the United States [46, 47]. In Jamaica, there is variability across sites, and triage may be performed by physicians and/or nurses. Not all doctors and nurses engaged in triage are trained in emergency medicine. Triage training is quite variable across the island [48, 49].

7.5 Use of technology to decrease wait time

The utilization of digital technology and simulation techniques seem to be promising strategies to decreasing waiting times. Studies have shown that applying agent-based model (ABM), queuing model (QM) and simulation techniques related to patient access and patient flow in the emergency room coupled with hospital information systems may be the answer for optimizing hospital processes and reducing bottlenecks in the ED [50, 51]. This is an area that is still evolving, but we believe it has enormous potential in reducing waiting times in the ED. Advance customer technologies empower individuals to manage their own time and optimize the queuing process with queue management software called Q-Flow that delivers next-generation customer experience and simple, effective queue management solutions [42, 52]. In countries such as the United Kingdom the use of patient safety tools that are provided by the NHS such as National Patient Safety Alerting System (NPSAS), which enables the dissemination of patient safety alerts to healthcare providers via a central alert system and a National Reporting and Learning System (NRLS) for reporting serious incidents, helped improve both patient safety and waiting time at the ED [42].

7.6 Health information exchange system, telemedicine and data protection management in Jamaica

Over the period of July 2012 to March 2013 Jamaica developed an integrated National Health Information System (NHISS) that supports timely and efficient data management. This system have helped to produce quality health information for evidence based decision making at all levels of the National Health System. The main aim of this NHISS is to improve the management of the healthcare system [43].

Jamaica is listed among 125 countries in the WHO Atlas of e-Health states in which e-Health strategies, such as policies, funding, capacity-building, and necessary legislative framework to protect patients' data, inter alia, are in place. In addition, it is mentioned the existence of telemedicine, mHealth, engagement of the population with social media, use of electronic records, use of e-learning in health sciences, and having a system in place to manage large amount of data [41]. The Electronic Management System in use in Jamaica is the first technology-driven element of its kind in Jamaica and the Caribbean region. It provides an electronic version of a patient's medical history, including demographics, progress notes, problems, medications, vital signs, past medical history, immunizations, laboratory data and radiology reports. The intention is to provide a complete and accurate summary of an individual's medical history that can be shared to improve the delivery of care and also provide quality data for decision-makers (health professionals, directors, researchers, citizens) across the health facilities of Jamaica [47].

7.7 Upgrading health policy for emergency care management

The main goal of safety and health programs is to prevent workplace injuries, illnesses, and deaths, as well as the suffering and financial hardship these events can cause for workers, their families, and employer especially for the emergency departments. The creation and recommended practices and policies, use a proactive approach to managing workplace safety and health, and upgrading is necessary. In Jamaica hospitals are some of the most frequented facilities based on the nature of the services they provide, and they are often overwhelmed with caring for and managing emergencies to reduce preventable mortality. Against this background, the Ministry of Health and Wellness normally request support from the Pan American Health Organization (PAHO), which facilitated an assessment through a survey and a two-day consensus meeting as part of an Emergency and Critical Care Assessment System. The PAHO governs the Caribbean Region and a similar approach in other Caribbean countries [42]. The Emergency and Critical Care Systems form an integral part of the broader implementation plan for the "Safe Systems Approach for Safer Roads in Jamaica," which sets the island on a path to achieve the goals proposed for the second Decade of Action for Road Safety 2021–2030. It also comprises all other types of injuries and critical illnesses requiring urgent medical attention and establishes the care all seriously ill patients should receive in every hospital [53]. Similarly, in their upgrade of health policies The NHS and UK Government have published a new two-year delivery plan today to help recover urgent and emergency care services, reduce waiting times, and improve patient experience. The plan focuses predominantly on the need to improve hospital discharge and join-up with adult social care, reflecting the challenges of an aging population and frailty. However, we know that children's urgent and emergency care has also faced unprecedented levels of demand and that some of the drivers of this are different than for adults. As part of the plan there are several welcome solutions to improve pediatric urgent and emergency care. These include: (1) expanding advice offered through NHS.UK and NHS111 online to support decision making for young people and families, including self-care and management, (2) roll out of acute pediatric respiratory hubs for children ahead of time for the winter, (3) expansion of virtual wards, with priority pathways for pediatrics, (4) expansion of virtual wards, with priority pathways for pediatrics, and (5) embedding family support workers in A & E settings to provide additional support to children and families presenting with non-urgent medical issues but overlapping needs [54].

7.8 Adequate evaluation process of risk management strategies

In Jamaica there is no documented established national plan for managing and evaluating emergency care risks. Therefore, the implementation of risk management strategies in emergency care at the public hospitals would be beneficial in maintaining patient safety in Jamaica [55]. However, there is a general national risk management policy that exists for the country governing all businesses [56]. Hence the importance of this study to aid in identifying the need for a national risk management policy specific for health care management. According to Gadding, to understand risk in the Emergency Department (ED), it is important to examine the workflow of the patient journey in an ED. The Emergency Department is a dynamic and often unpredictable place, which makes it a high-risk inducing environment. The staff of an ED may see anything during a shift, ranging from a common cold or upset stomach that are treated with a simple medication to a trauma or cardiac arrest that requires full resuscitation efforts. Speed, efficiency, and accuracy of assessing, diagnosing, and treating patients are essential, due to the unpredictable and often heavy flow of patients through an ED. A visit to an ED involves a complex series of decisions, interactions, and activities, which will make it vital for risk planning and assessment to be accurate. A systematic approach that facilitates fast, efficient, and accurate patient documentation and treatment within defined processes is required to minimize unexpected failures or human errors [32]. The main objective of carrying out the process of management of risk is appropriately controlling the health variables which affect the overall health condition of patients for enhancing the potential of achieving the most appropriate outcomes. Since the main reasons for accidents happening are a set of known or unknown failures in the health care system, in this regard conducting standardized approaches for the management of risks in a hierarchical framework could be very effective [57]. Moreover, preparing more accurate and standardized plans which sufficiently are investigated and prepared with continuous monitoring could be very effective in ensuring the proper management of the potential risks and damages to the patients and the emergency staff. The precise implementation of these kinds of strategies is strongly associated with the involvement of patients and the emergency staff and the overall support of administrative and Insurance organizations [58].

7.9 Decreasing overcrowding in A & Es

Empirical studies have demonstrated that overcrowding is a major risk factor to patient safety and mortality in emergency rooms worldwide. Addressing this problem has been a major challenge in emergency care for many years [58, 59]. Despite the existence of multiple interventions to address this problem, it continues to spiral out of control in many countries including Jamaica. Therefore, it is important that each healthcare system has consistent ongoing review of existing management of the influx of patients into emergency rooms. This influx may be seasonal or situational and so plans should be put in place to address the unavoidable increase in patient load. Where patients can be seen at clinics, private hospitals or medical offices they should be encouraged to do so [60, 61].

However, preventing the influx of patients in emergency rooms does not alter how patients receive emergency care. Therefore, it is essential that the emergency care provided to patients is efficient in decreasing long wait time as well. Interventions that can be employed to improve wait time in the Jamaican public emergency setting include improving hospital capacity, decreasing overcrowding by using observation units as a component of the triage process [62, 63].

8. Conclusion

The growing problem of long wait time in the public hospitals is not a unique phenomenon but is a global health care concern with multiple contributing factors. Therefore, there is no one solution that can be employed to adequately address the health care dilemma. However, the use of a risk management approach to addressing the health care issue is highly recommended since it allows for advance planning, implementation of interventions and the evaluation of outcomes to mitigate or prevent major challenges that could negatively impact patient safety in emergency care management. Other important measures that can be taken include ongoing upgrade of national health policy in emergency care management, improving triage systems, decreasing overcrowding and the adequate use of modern technology to decrease wait time for patients to receive effective and efficient emergency health care. To achieve this feat a collaborative approach must be engaged including the involvement of the government's public and private health care systems.

In conclusion, further studies should be done in identifying the main risk factors that contributes to the long wait time at hospitals in Jamaica. Thus, creating the opportunity for the development of universal health care policies to effectively decrease long wait time in emergency rooms in public hospitals, by employing risk management strategies.

Acknowledgements

I would first like to thank God for giving me the opportunity to complete this project with much success. I am also grateful for the support provided by the leadership and management of the Brown's Town Community College in St. Ann, Jamaica in the completion of this invaluable research work to improve health care practice on a global scale. I would also like to thank all the institutions that have contributed to my academic growth over the years. More so, I want to thank IntechOpen for the confidence placed in me to take on such a major project for the first time in coauthoring in a book through a globally renown journal. I am forever grateful and do anticipate further collaboration of this nature and magnitude in the future.

Funding

No funding was solicited for this project.

Conflicts of interest

The authors confirm that this chapter content has no conflict of interest.

Author details

Opal Davidson[1*], James Fallah[2], Denice Curtis[3] and Chukwuma Richard Uzoka[4]

1 Browns Town Community College, Brown's Town, Jamaica

2 Northern Caribbean University, Mandeville, Jamaica

3 Massachusetts College of Pharmacy and Health Sciences, USA

4 Acclaimed Global Health Institute, Beverley, Jamaica

*Address all correspondence to: opaldon6@yahoo.com

IntechOpen

© 2024 The Author(s). Licensee IntechOpen. This chapter is distributed under the terms of the Creative Commons Attribution License (http://creativecommons.org/licenses/by/3.0), which permits unrestricted use, distribution, and reproduction in any medium, provided the original work is properly cited.

References

[1] Biya M, Gezahagn M, Birhanu B, et al. Waiting time and its associated factors in patients presenting to outpatient departments at Public Hospitals of Jimma Zone, Southwest Ethiopia. BMC Health Services Research. 2022;**22**:107. DOI: 10.1186/s12913-022-07502-8

[2] Gertz AH, Pollack CC, Schultheiss MD, Brownstein JS. Delayed medical care and underlying health in the United States during the COVID-19 pandemic: A cross-sectional study. Preventive Medical Reports. 2022;**28**:101882. DOI: 10.1016/j.pmedr.2022.101882. Epub 2022 Jul 5

[3] Lasater KB, Sloane DM, McHugh MD, Cimiotti JP, Riman KA, Martin B, et al. Evaluation of hospital nurse-to-patient staffing ratios and sepsis bundles on patient outcomes. American Journal of Infection Control. 2021;**49**(7):868-873. DOI: 10.1016/j.ajic.2020.12.002. Epub 2020 Dec 10

[4] Ackroyd-Stolarz S, Guernsey J, Mackinnon N, Kovacs G. The association between a prolonged stay in the emergency department and adverse events in older patients. 2011

[5] Girvan, T. Waiting in Vain? Understanding Emergency Room Priority Levels [Internet]. 2023. Available from: https://www.jamaicaobserver.com/health/waiting-in-vain-4/ [Accessed: January 05, 2024]

[6] Coombs, M. Universal Coverage in Jamaica [Internet] 2012. Available from: https://www3.paho.org/hq/dmdocuments/2012/COOMBS-JAM-BAR-22oct2012.pdf [Accessed: January 05, 2024]

[7] Thomas C. Hospital Managers Urged to Ease Wait Times [Internet] 2021. Available from: https://jamaica-gleaner.com/article/lead-stories/20210609/hospital-managers-urged-ease-wait-times [Accessed: January 05, 2024]

[8] Small, S. COVID-19 Cases Still on the Rise [Internet]. 2023. Available from: https://jamaica-gleaner.com/article/news/20230719/covid-19-cases-still-rise [Accessed: January 05, 2024]

[9] Emanuel L, Berwick D, Conway J, et al. What exactly is patient safety? In: Henriksen K, Battles JB, Keyes MA, et al., editors. Advances in Patient Safety: New Directions and Alternative Approaches, Assessment. Vol. 1. Rockville (MD): Agency for Healthcare Research and Quality; 2008. Available from: https://www.ncbi.nlm.nih.gov/books/NBK43629/2

[10] Ackroyd-Stolarz S, Guernsey J, MacKinnon N, Kovacs G. The association between a prolonged stay in the emergency department and adverse events in older patients admitted to hospital: A retrospective cohort study. BMJ Quality & Safety. 2011;**20**:564-569. DOI: 10.1136/bmjqs.2009.034926

[11] BMJ-British Medical Journal. Long emergency waiting times linked to increased risk of adverse events. ScienceDaily. 1 June 2011. Available from: www.sciencedaily.com/releases/2011/06/110601204048.htm

[12] Nyce A, Gandhi S, Freeze B, Bosire J, Ricca T, Kupersmith E, et al. Association of emergency department waiting times with patient experience in admitted and discharged patients. Journal of Patient Experience. 2021;**8**:23743735211011404. DOI: 10.1177/23743735211011404

[13] Khankeh HR, Khorasani-Zavareh D, Azizi-Naghdloo F, Hoseini MA,

Rahgozar M. Triage effect on wait time of receiving treatment services and patients satisfaction in the emergency department: Example from Iran. Iranian Journal of Nursing and Midwifery Research. 2013;**18**(1):79-83

[14] Goodacre S, Webster A. Who waits longest in the emergency department and who leaves without being seen? Emergency Medicine Journal. 2005;**22**:93-96

[15] Savioli G, Ceresa IF, Gri N, Bavestrello Piccini G, Longhitano Y, Zanza C, et al. Emergency department overcrowding: Understanding the factors to find corresponding solutions. Journal of Personalized Medicine. 2022;**12**(2):279. DOI: 10.3390/jpm12020279

[16] Moskowitz, D. The Importance of Health Care Risk Management [Internet]. 2022. Available from: https://www.investopedia.com/articles/personal-finance/072315/importance-healthcare-risk-management.asp#:~:text=Risk%20management%20is%20the%20process,makes%20the%20stakes%20significantly%20higher [Accessed: January 05, 2024]

[17] World Health Organization. Global Patient Safety Action Plan [Internet]. 2023. Available from: https://www.who.int/teams/integrated-health-services/patient-safety/policy/global-patient-safety-action-plan [Accessed: January 05, 2024]

[18] O'Cathain A, Croot L, Duncan E, Rousseau N, Sworn K, Turner KM, et al. Guidance on how to develop complex interventions to improve health and healthcare. BMJ Open. 2019;**9**(8):e029954. DOI: 10.1136/bmjopen-2019-029954

[19] Clarke GM, Conti S, Wolters AT, Steventon A. Evaluating the impact of healthcare interventions using routine data. BMJ. 2019;**365**:l2239. DOI: 10.1136/bmj.l2239

[20] Kahraman J. Europe's Hospitals in the Spotlight – A Journey Through 5 Regions [Internet]. 2023. Available from: https://www.swisslog-healthcare.com/en-gb/company/blog/europes-hospitals-in-the-spotlight [Accessed: January 07, 2024]

[21] Watt E. Risk management planning. In: Project Management for Skills for All Careers, Chapter 16 by Project Management Open Resources and TAP-a-PM. 2nd ed. Available from: https://opentextbc.ca/projectmanagement/chapter/chapter-16-risk-management-planning-project-management/

[22] OECD. Healthcare wait Times by Country 2024 [Internet]. 2024. Available from: https://worldpopulationreview.com/country-rankings/health-care-wait-times-by-country [Accessed: January 05, 2024]

[23] Schut F, Varkevisser M. The Netherlands. In: Siciliani L, Borowitz M, Moran V, editors. Waiting Time Policies in the Health Sector: What Works? Paris: OECD Publishing; 2013. DOI: 10.1787/9789264179080-13-en

[24] Campbell D, Duncan P. One in 10 A & E patients in England face 'dangerous' 12 hour waits. The Guardian [Internet]. 2023. Available from: https://www.theguardian.com/society/2023/apr/13/accident-emergency-patients-nhs-england-dangerous-wait-times-12-hours Accessed: January 09, 2024

[25] Nuffield Trust & the Health Foundation. UK Long Wait Time Statistics [Internet]. 2023. Available from: https://www.nuffieldtrust.org.uk/resource/a-e-waiting-times [Accessed: January 05, 2024]

[26] Lakeridge Health Department. Emergency Department Wait Times [Internet]. 2023. Available from: https://www.lakeridgehealth.on.ca/en/ourservices/emergency-department-wait-times.asp [Accessed: January 05, 2024]

[27] Heilman JA, Tanski M, Burns B, Lin A, Ma J. Decreasing time to pain relief for emergency department patients with extremity fractures. BMJ Quality Improvement Reports. 2016;**5**(1):u209522.w7251. DOI: 10.1136/bmjquality.u209522.w7251

[28] Baker DW, Stevens CD, Brook RH. Patients who leave a public hospital emergency department without being seen by a physician: Causes and consequences. Journal of the American Medical Association. 1991;**266**(8):1085-1090. DOI: 10.1001/jama.1991.03470080055029

[29] Yuzeng S, Hui LL. Improving the wait time to triage at the emergency department. BMJ Open Quality. 2020;**9**(1):e000708. DOI: 10.1136/bmjoq-2019-000708

[30] Willcox S, Seddon M, Dunn S, Edwards R, Pearse J, Tu J. Measuring and reducing waiting times: A cross-national comparison of strategies. Health Affairs (Project Hope). 2007;**26**:1078-1087. DOI: 10.1377/hlthaff.26.4.1078

[31] De Freitas L, Goodacre S, O'Hara R, Thokala P, Hariharan S. Qualitative exploration of patient flow in a Caribbean emergency department. BMJ Open. 2020;**10**(12):e041422. DOI: 10.1136/bmjopen-2020-041422

[32] Edwards M, Cooper A, Hughes T, Davies F, Price D, Anderson P, et al. The effectiveness of primary care streaming in emergency departments on decision-making and patient flow and safety - A realist evaluation. International Emergency Nursing. 2022;**62**:101155. DOI: 10.1016/j.ienj.2022.101155. Epub 2022 Mar 23

[33] Barbados Today. Public Notice: Increased wait times at the Accident and Emergency Department [Internet]. Available from: https://barbadostoday.bb/2023/11/01/public-notice-increased-wait-times-at-the-accident-and-emergency-department/ [Accessed: January 05, 2024]

[34] Lee J, Yoon S. Nature and patient waiting: Mediating effects of anxiety and perceived wait time on the association between nature and service perception. Journal of Environmental Psychology. 2023;**91**:102113. DOI: 10.1016/j.jenvp.2023.102113. ISSN 0272-4944. Available from: https://www.sciencedirect.com/science/article/pii/S0272494423001615

[35] Pearlmutter MD, Dwyer KH, Burke LG, Rathlev N, Maranda L, Volturo G. Analysis of emergency department length of stay for mental health patients at ten Massachusetts Emergency Departments. Annals of Emergency Medicine. 2017;**70**(2):193-202.e16. DOI: 10.1016/j.annemergmed.2016.10.005. Epub 2017 Jan 4

[36] Fitzgerald G, Jelinek G, Scott D, Gerdtz MF. Emergency department triage revisited. Emergency Medicine Journal. 2010;**27**(2):86-92

[37] Moskop, Iserson. Triage in medicine, part II: Underlying values and principles. Annals of Emergency Medicine. 2007;**49**(3):282-287

[38] Aacharya RP, Gastmans C, Denier Y. Emergency department triage: An ethical analysis. BMC Emergency Medicine. 2011;**11**:16. DOI: 10.1186/1471-227X-11-16

[39] French S, Gordon-Strachan G, Kerr K, Bisasor-McKenzie J, Innis L, Tanabe P. Implementing the emergency severity index triage system in Jamaican accident and emergency departments. Journal of Emergency Nursing. 2019;**45**(2):124-131. DOI: 10.1016/j.jen.2018.11.010. Epub 2018 Dec 24

[40] ACF-technologies. Patient Experience: 8 Effective Ways to Reduce Wait Times and Save Money [Internet]. 2023. Available from: https://www.acftechnologies.com/blog/8-effective-ways-to-reduce-patient-wait-times/ [Accessed: January 05, 2024]

[41] Shen Y, Lee LH. Improving the wait time to consultation at the emergency department. BMJ Open Quality. 2018;7(1):e000131. DOI: 10.1136/bmjoq-2017-000131

[42] French S, Gordon-Strachan G, Kerr K, Bisasor-McKenzie J, Innis L, Tanabe P. Assessment of interrater reliability of the emergency severity index after implementation in emergency departments in Jamaica using a learning collaborative approach. Journal of Emergency Nursing. 2021;**47**(1):58-65. ISSN 0099-1767. DOI: 10.1016/j.jen.2020.07.003

[43] Campbell, A. e-Health in the J'can Public Health System: Where are We? The Jamaican Observer [Internet]. 2018. Available from: https://www.jamaicaobserver.com/columns/e-health-in-the-jcan-public-health-system-where-are-we/ [Accessed: January 16, 2024]

[44] Yancey CC, O'Rourke MC. Emergency Department Triage [Updated 2023 Aug 28]. In: StatPearls [Internet]. Treasure Island (FL): StatPearls Publishing; 2023. Available from: https://www.ncbi.nlm.nih.gov/books/NBK557583/

[45] Ministry of Health Jamaica. National Health Information System Strengthening and e-Health Strategic Plan 2014 to 2018 [Internet]. 2013. Available from: https://www.moh.gov.jm/wp-content/uploads/2015/07/MOH_NHIS-eHealth_StrategicPlanFINAL.pdf

[46] NHS. Our National Patient Safety Alerts [Internet]. 2012. Available from: https://www.england.nhs.uk/patient-safety/patient-safety-insight/patient-safety-alerts/ [Accessed: January 05, 2024]

[47] Singer SJ, Benzer JK, Hamdan SU. Improving health care quality and safety: The role of collective learning. Journal of Healthcare Leadership. 2015;**7**:91-107. DOI: 10.2147/JHL.S70115

[48] Laskowski M, McLeod RD, Friesen MR, Podaima BW, Alfa AS. Models of emergency departments for reducing patient waiting times. PLoS One. 2009;**4**(7):e6127. DOI: 10.1371/journal.pone.0006127

[49] Ahmad J, Iqbal J, Ahmad I, Khan ZA, Tiwana MI, Khan K. A simulation based study for managing hospital resources by reducing patient waiting time. IEEE Access. 2020;**8**:193523-193531. DOI: 10.1109/ACCESS.2020.3032760

[50] Heslin SM, Nappi M, Kelly G, et al. Rapid creation of an emergency department telehealth program during the COVID-19 pandemic. Journal of Telemedicine and Telecare. 2022;**28**(3):207-212. DOI: 10.1177/1357633X20952632

[51] Q-nomy Health Care Solutions. Complete Patient Flow Management Simplifies Dependency [Internet]. 2022. Available from: https://www.qnomyhealth.com/emergency-departments#:~:text=The%20

Q%2Dflow%20platform%20
offers,patients%20visit%20the%20
ER%2FED [Accessed: December 29, 2023]

[52] Stavropoulou C, Doherty C, Tosey P. How effective are incident-reporting systems for improving patient safety? A systematic literature review. Milbank Quarterly. 2015;**93**(4):826-866. DOI: 10.1111/1468-0009.12166

[53] PAHO. PAHO Facilitates Assessment of Jamaica's Emergency and Critical Care System During 2-Day Consensus Meeting [Internet]. 2023. Available from: https://www.paho.org/en/news/13-9-2023-paho-facilitates-assessment-jamaicas-emergency-and-critical-care-system-during-2-day [Accessed: January 16, 2024]

[54] Royal College of Paediatrics and child health. The NHS and UK Government have Published a New Two-year Delivery Plan Today to Help Recover Urgent and Emergency Care Services, Reduce Waiting Times, and Improve Patient Experience [Internet]. 2023. Available from: https://www.rcpch.ac.uk/news-events/news/nhs-englands-plan-recover-urgent-emergency-care-services [Accessed: January 16, 2024]

[55] Gadding MA. Risk Management in the Emergency Department. Omnia Health [Internet]. 2019. Available from: https://insights.omnia-health.com/medical-specialities/risk-management-emergency-department [Accessed: January 07, 2024]

[56] Tavirani MR, Beigvand HH. A review of various methods of management of risk in the field of emergency medicine. Open Access Macedonian Journal of Medical Sciences. 2019;**7**(23):4179-4187. DOI: 10.3889/oamjms.2019.616

[57] Krist AH, Tong ST, Aycock RA, Longo DR. Engaging patients in decision-making and behavior change to promote prevention. Studies in Health Technology and Informatics. 2017;**240**:284-302

[58] Sachs CJ, Yu CK, Nauka PC, Schriger DL. Systems opportunities to reduce ED crowding from nonemergency referrals. American Journal of Medical Quality. 2018;**33**(1):37-42. DOI: 10.1177/1062860617700721

[59] Pines JM, Hilton JA, Weber EJ, Alkemade AJ, Al Shabanah H, Anderson PD, et al. International perspectives on emergency department crowding. Academic Emergency Medicine. 2011;**18**(12):1358-1370. DOI: 10.1111/j.1553-2712.2011.01235.x

[60] Coster JE, Turner JK, Bradbury D, Cantrell A. Why do people choose emergency and urgent care services? A rapid review utilizing a systematic literature search and narrative synthesis. Academic Emergency Medicine. 2017;**24**(9):1137-1149. DOI: 10.1111/acem.13220

[61] Henry, O. Increased Patient Visits to Health Centres Under Reducing Waiting Time Initiative [Internet]. 2019. Available from: https://jis.gov.jm/features/increased-patient-visits-to-health-centres-under-reducing-waiting-time-initiative/#:~:text=She%20notes%20
that%20patients%20will%20be%20
encouraged%20to,for%20visits%20
to%20the%20emergency%20room%20
and%20hospitalisation [Accessed: January 18, 2024]

[62] Viccellio P, Hochman KA, Semczuk P, Santora C. Right focus, right solution: How reducing variability in admission and discharge improves hospital capacity and flow. In: Litvak E, editor. Optimizing Patient Flow: Advanced Strategies for Managing Variability to Enhance Access, Quality,

and Safety. Oak Brook, IL: The Joint Commission; 2018. pp. 97-112

[63] Baugh CW, Venkatesh AK, Bohan JS. Emergency department observation units: A clinical and financial benefit for hospitals. Health Care Management Review. 2011;**36**(1):28-37. DOI: 10.1097/HMR.0b013e3181f3c035

Chapter 8

Does Social Media Promote Health Misinformation? The Malaysian Scenario

Nazri Nordin

Abstract

In Malaysia, social media such as MySpace, Twitter, LinkedIn, Flickr, Tumblr, Wikipedia, YouTube, Google Plus, and Facebook are the cheapest and easiest media platforms for consumers to access health information. In social media, the audiences will be presented with information on how to make self-diagnosis and select health products to treat their undesirable medical conditions. However, studies demonstrated the potential of social media to mislead audiences into believing that health products are safe and cost-effective. In contrast, the consumers might potentially encounter unwanted adverse drug events. It is even worse when the consumers experience emotional disturbance, financial loss, and physical damage. Therefore, this article will highlight the negative effect of social media on the healthcare system by pointing out an example of *Nigella sativa*. Hopefully, this article will alert the authorities to monitor social media for misleading health information.

Keywords: social media, marketers, black seed, health products, *Nigella sativa*, misinformation, undesirable effect, drug-related problems, STARZ-DRP

1. Introduction

Social media such as MySpace, Twitter, LinkedIn, Pinterest, Flickr, Tumblr, Wikipedia, YouTube, Google Plus, and Facebook are most accessible platforms for seeking information about health products [1]. Social media is rapidly emerging as a powerful tool to establish strong trustworthiness and connection between marketers and audiences. It allows marketers to educate their audiences about health information as well as promote products [2]. Most of the time, marketers succeed in attaining their audiences' reliability, truth, or ability to accept the truth about their speech or writing [3]. Unfortunately, social media might not have a precise unit or division to enforce legal action toward marketers' misbehaviors [4]. It is crucial to form a legal advocacy organization to guarantee that marketers comply with domestic laws regarding medicine and cosmetic advertisements. Alternatively, the marketers may present or claim untrustworthy information that might potentially lead to health misinformation [1].

Marketers usually include individuals, entrepreneurs, or healthcare practitioners. Each marketer has distinct characteristics, knowledge, and skills. For example,

IntechOpen

individuals and entrepreneurs are not trained to act, behave, or conduct themselves according to medical practice. They do not attend any formal long-term course that can prepare them with knowledge and skills for advocating, educating, or responding to a particular medical disease. Therefore, they always assign someone to express ideas or feelings about health products on social media. The assignee shall reveal his or her experience of being healthier after consuming the product [5–7]. For that reason, he or she recommends that audiences buy and consume a similar product. Most of the time, the assignee shall not reveal undesirable experiences after consuming the product.

Therefore, the majority of them consistently provide proof of the safe usage and performance of their goods by emphasizing testimonials from customers who are familiar with the items. Entrepreneurs may designate someone to arrange a personal interview with an individual who may inform audiences about their experience and satisfaction with the items. Prior to being shared on social media, the entire interview session must be accurately documented. Typically, the interview process does not uncover negative events. The lack of training among entrepreneurs in assessing, analyzing, and reporting side effects or adverse pharmacological responses experienced by their clients is the reason for this.

Physicians or pharmacists are well-trained to act, behave, or conduct themselves in response to a specific medical condition and medication use. Their knowledge and skills had been evaluated appropriately during their long-term university course. Therefore, they can advocate for their audiences about medical conditions and medication selections. Nonetheless, it is essential to monitor potential unethical marketing conduct among physicians and pharmacists [8]. They have the ability to quickly earn the trust of the audience, who rely on them to use their words and writing responsibly [9]. Consequently, they may inadvertently deceive the audience into believing that their items for sale are the most superior or sought-after or quality in demand [10]. Such unethical actions will harm the reputation of the healthcare profession [11].

In Malaysia, there are a few articles that point out some health misinformation issues, particularly related to breast cancer prevention and treatment [12], vaccines [13, 14], smoking [15], and medicine [16]. However, the author could not find any article that highlights misinformation about health products on social media. The previous study showed that Twitter had a higher prevalence of health misinformation compared to other social media platforms [10]. Generally, the previous articles on social media have identified health misinformation pertaining to smoking goods [17–19], vaccines [20–22], diseases [23–25], and treatments [26, 27]. In the realm of social media, the dissemination of health misinformation, disinformation, or false news is more prevalent and widespread than the dissemination of scientific facts and data [28, 29]. Presenting such information in simple language is to facilitate audience comprehension. In addition, individuals with varying educational backgrounds may not possess knowledge of scientific and technical vocabulary, including words, concepts, formulae, and symbols that are widely comprehended by scientists [28, 29]. Consequently, viewers are more inclined to evaluate unscientific social media platforms for information. A number of studies in Malaysia highlight health misinformation concerns, namely breast cancer prevention and treatment [12], vaccines [13, 14], smoking [15], and medication [16]. Unfortunately, the author was unable to locate any articles that specifically address the dissemination of false or misleading information on health items on social media platforms.

In Malaysia, health products are registered under natural or traditional products or health supplements [30]. The National Pharmaceutical Regulatory Agency (NPRA) is a legal authority that organizes and approves product registrations [31]. During the application process, the applicants need to submit to NPRA a list of documents, such as a good manufacturing practice certificate, as well as quality, safety, and efficacy documents, respectively [32, 33]. Based on the documentation, NPRA shall analyze it in detail before assigning a unique, valid registration number for the product. Such registration numbers shall begin with "MAL," followed by 8-digit numbers and end with an alphabet to indicate their registration category, which is "T" for natural or traditional products and "N" for health supplements [31]. The main reason for the registration number is to ease NPRA in monitoring the distribution of the products in the domestic market. Nonetheless, during the registration process, NPRA might not discover or identify the presence or existence of undesirable effects of the product unless the consumers report their experience about such adverse drug events to physicians or pharmacists. Therefore, NPRA has established a form to be filled out by the physician or pharmacist if they find potential or actual adverse drug reactions [34]. It reflects that the health care system requires physicians and pharmacists to identify, prevent, and monitor undesirable effects of health products. For that reason, physicians and pharmacists must know about each product and be alert of unwanted effects their patients might encounter after consuming it.

Nigella sativa (*Habbatus Sauda*), known as black seed, is commonly consumed by the Malay people in Malaysia. In general, people consume black seed as a daily basic supplement because they believe it can help them be healthier [35]. Social media highlights the black seed's advantages to emphasize their possible negative pharmacological reactions. Hence, this chapter will specifically examine the black seed to ascertain any possible dissemination of inaccurate health information and its impact on the liver. This article aims to raise awareness among authorities regarding the dissemination of disinformation concerning black seed on social media.

2. Materials and methods

Searching for some information about black seed and its advertisements was performed by assessing Google and YouTube, respectively. Such activities paid particular attention to articles and advertisements published from January 1, 2014, till December 31, 2023. The keywords used to search were *Nigella sativa*, black seed, contents, active ingredients, liver disorders, advertisement, benefits, harmful, unwanted effects, side effects, adverse drug events, undesirable effects, pharmacological, toxicological properties, oral consumption, and cautions. In addition, the author highlights a few cases that were noted in actual practice regarding the potential undesirable effects of black seed on the liver.

3. Results

3.1 *Nigella sativa*

Nigella sativa, or black seed, originates from the Ranunculacea family [36]. *Nigella sativa* contains thymoquinone (TQ), alkaloids (nigellicines and nigelledine), saponins (alpha-hederin), flavonoids, proteins, fatty acids, and many others [37, 38]. Nonetheless, TQ is the black seed's most abundant constituent or predominant active lipophilic component. Therefore, the black seed has some therapeutic effects, such as antiproliferation, apoptosis induction, cell cycle arrest, reactive oxygen species generation, and antimetastasis [39]. However, its effectiveness and oral bioavailability are limited by its lipophilicity and poor solubility in water [40, 41]. As a result, the black seed might potentially induce unwanted adverse effects. For example, a previous finding noted that the consumption of black seed in the form of oil and crushed seed demonstrated significant increases in the readings of liver markers, which are alanine transaminase (ALT) [42], alkaline phosphatase (ALP) [43], gamma-glutamyltransferase (GGT) [42], and aspartate transaminase (AST) [42, 43]. Another study found that nasal drops containing black seed oil increased significantly in AST and ALT [44].

Most previous studies assessed ALT, ALP, AST, and GGT among the participants who consumed black seed for less than 3 months [45–48]. It is noted that the outcomes of the studies demonstrated desirable effects on liver function. Nonetheless, it is believed that prolonged exposure to TQ might result in toxicity to the biological body system [49, 50]. TQ might also have an undesirable drug interaction with other medications [51, 52]. TQ in black seed oil is well tolerated at a dose from 75 to 2600 mg/day or less than 2% with no toxicity to observe [53]. TQ is metabolized in the liver into thymohydroquinone [54]. In a previous study, following oral administration of TQ in animal models, the half-life (T1/2) was about 276.61 ± 8.48 minutes [55]. The estimated percentage of TQ-protein binding in human plasma is about 98.99% [56]. For that reason, it is believed that long-term consumption of *Nigella sativa* will lead consumers to undesirable medical conditions. A case study report of acute renal failure had been associated with 2–2.5 grams of *Nigella sativa* capsules daily for 6 days in a diabetic patient [57].

In actual practice, the author reported the occurrence of liver diseases resulting from the possible consumption of black seed.

3.2 Advertisements on YouTube

The data indicated that marketers on social media have been informing the audiences about the advantages of black seed. Black seed has been hailed as a miraculous natural remedy for treating several medical conditions, including diabetes [58–62], liver [59, 60], kidney [60], alopecia [61], cancer [60–65], cardiovascular disease [58–62], central nervous system [59, 62], hyperlipidemia [59–61], man infertility [60, 61], libido [60], liver [60], menstrual pain [60], seizure [58], stomach [58–60, 64], asthma [59, 60, 65, 66], fibroid [66], immune system [58, 61, 62, 64, 65], parasites [60], fungal [58], human immunodeficiency virus [61], staphylococcus [61], tuberculosis [61], influenza [61], gonorrhea [61], candida [61], malaria [61], obesity [58, 61], and arthritis [62, 64, 65]. Several marketers contended that including black seed in one's diet is a suitable means of achieving proper nutritional intake. However, the data also indicated that there were marketers who advised their audiences to visit their physicians for an appropriate dosage regimen prior to taking the black seed [62, 67]. Apart from that, some marketers were found to be educating their audiences about the safe use of black seed [59–61, 63].

4. Discussion

In Malaysia, black seed is controlled by the Food Safety and Quality Division, Ministry of Health. Food and drink supplement products are not allowed to make any medicinal claim. Such claims include, for example, that black seed is able to enhance men's sexual drive, can induce weight loss, and treats kidney, cancer, seizure, venereal and cardiovascular diseases. Without such a claim, marketers are free to promote, market, and distribute black seed on social media. However, the potential for health misinformation about black seeds on social media still exists [68]. For example, black seed was described as a potential supplement to treat asthmatic patients even though the promotion content was inconsistent with the Global Initiative for Asthma 2019 guidelines [68]. For that reason, it is essential to control advertising activities on social media [1]. In Malaysia, any individual who advertises a product without permission from the legal authority can be fined up to a maximum of RM3,000 or a jail sentence not exceeding 1 year or both for the first offense and for a subsequent offense, a fine up to a maximum of RM5,000 or a jail sentence not exceeding 2 years or both [69]. The Medicines (Advertisement and Sale) Act of 1956 regulates individuals' actions to prevent them from misleading their audiences [70].

Medicines (Advertisement and Sale) Act 1956 highlights that individuals cannot mislead people into believing and consuming a specific product to treat a specific medical disease [70]. Marketers are prohibited from advertising their products as effective in preventing or treating ailments, such as kidney failure, heart disease, diabetes, epilepsy or fits, paralysis, tuberculosis, asthma, leprosy, cancer, deafness, drug addiction, hernia or rupture, diseases of the eye, hypertension, mental disorder, infertility, frigidity, impairment of sexual function or impotence venereal disease, and nervous debility, or other complaint or infirmity, arising from or relating to sexual intercourse [70]. However, marketers from other countries are not bound by Malaysian law. For that reason, they continue to promote their products on social media to attract audiences' attention [71–73]. It is even worse when Malaysian marketers promote their products on social media managed by other countries [74–76]. Consequently, the Malaysian government may face several obstacles in pursuing legal action against the marketers.

Most studies focused on the benefits of black seed instead of its unwanted effects. They were designed to investigate the positive impact of black seed toward health within 3 months. In addition, participants must adhere to the inclusion and exclusion criteria prior to the studies. A control group of health participants involved in such studies might not represent the actual scenario in practice. Therefore, most of the studies might not capture the incidence of unwanted effects. However, physicians and pharmacists in their line of work have the opportunity to inform patients about the adverse consequences of black seed. For instance, the author can identify such adverse consequences due to patients ingesting the black seed in an unregulated environment (see **Tables 1**–5).

It is believed that the consumption of black seed can cause potential liver disorders. High readings of AST, ALP, ALP, and GGT reflect potential liver disorders, as depicted in **Tables 1**–5. A cross-reference to investigate the incidence of liver disorders also showed that black seed can cause medical conditions, as shown in previous reported studies [42–44]. Therefore, it is essential to determine if the customers are suitable candidates to consume black seed. It is because black seed is also not suitable for an individual who has specific medical conditions such as hypoglycemia [77], bleeding [78], and hypotension [79]. In addition, black seed might also potentially cause soft-tissue damage [80] due to the increased number of LDH (see **Tables 1**, **4**, and 5) and CRP (see **Tables 4** and 5). Nonetheless, these findings require further studies. Currently, physicians and chemists need to thoroughly evaluate their clients' medical and prescription histories to determine if they are appropriate candidates for consuming black seed. The reason is that each client has a unique pathophysiology. These variances necessitate a distinct approach to therapy. For instance, a client with profuse

A female patient, who is 56 years old, complained of unresolved vertigo. She did not consume any medication but the black seed for the past 1 year to treat the vertigo. She was not able to tell the exact strength of the black seed. An earlier laboratory test demonstrated the following abnormal readings, which were erythrocyte sedimentation rate (ESR) = 67.0 mm/hr., hemoglobin (Hb) = 12.8 g/dL, mean corpuscular hemoglobin concentration (MCHC) = 31 g/dL, neutrophil = 76%, fasting blood sugar (FBS) = 6.5 mmol/L, total cholesterol = 6.2 mmol/L, low-density lipoprotein (LDL) = 3.8 mmol/L, ALP = 125 U/L, AST = 73 U/L, ALT = 100 U/L, and lactate dehydrogenase (LDH) = 246 U/L. The author noted that the black seed could be the risk factor for the incidence of liver disorders. Therefore, the patient was advised to stop consuming the black seed. After 6 months, a post-laboratory test demonstrated the following readings, which were ESR = 37.0 mm/hr., hemoglobin = 11.0 g/dL, PCV = 35%, MCHC = 32 g/dL, neutrophil = 45.9%, fasting blood sugar = 5.2 mmol/L, total cholesterol = 5.1 mmol/L, LDL = 3.1 mmol/L, ALP = 144 U/L, AST = 14 U/L, ALT = 13 U/L, and LDH = 222 U/L.

Table 1.
Case # 1.

A male patient, 56 years old, complained of uncontrolled blood glucose. The patient had been diagnosed with diabetes mellitus type 2 for the past 7 years, but he refused to consume the prescribed medication to control his blood glucose. Instead, he constantly consumed the black seed for the past 3 years to eliminate the disease. A pre-laboratory test showed the following abnormal readings which were ESR = 13 mm/hr., platelet count = 146 x 10^9/L, eosinophil = 10.7, FBS = 23.8 mmol/L, glycosylated hemoglobin (HbA1C) = 13.3% (122 mmol/mol), LDL = 2.8 mmol/l, AST = 92 u/L, ALT = 205 u/L, GGT = 98 iu/L, thyroid stimulating hormone (TSH) = 0.32. Such results indicated that the black seed might cause a potential risk of liver disorders. Therefore, the patient was advised to stop the consumption of black seed. However, the patient failed to attend the follow-up monitoring session after 6 months. As a result, the latest laboratory test is lacking.

Table 2.
Case # 2

A male patient, 66 years old, complained of unresolved gouty arthritis. He had been diagnosed with gouty arthritis for the past 2 months. In addition, he was also diagnosed with obsessive-compulsive drugs and prescribed clonazepam 0.5 mg and fluvoxamine Maleate 50 mg. He also constantly consumed black seed for the past 2 months to eliminate gouty arthritis. Pre-laboratory test demonstrated the following abnormal readings which were Hb = 19 g/dL, red cell distribution width (RDW) = 14.5%, packed cell volume (PCV) = 58, ESR = 41 mm/hr., uric acid (UA) = 0.59 mmol/L, phosphate = 0.79 mmol/L, GGT = 83 U/L, total cholesterol = 5.6 mmol/L, high-density lipoprotein (HDL) = 0.9 mmol/L, LDL = 3.4 mmol/L, triglycerides = 2.8 mmol/L, and HbA1C = 6.5% (48 mmol/mol). Results from the test demonstrated that he potentially has a mild liver disorder due to the consumption of black seed. Therefore, the patient was advised to stop the consumption of the black seed, and he was advised to consume milk thistle 200 mg twice daily for 6 months. A post-laboratory test demonstrated the following readings which were Hb = 17.1 g/dL, RDW = 14.0%, PCV = 52, ESR = 43 mm/hr., UA = 0.45 mmol/L, GGT = 40 U/L, total cholesterol = 3.4 mmol/L, HDL = 0.9 mmol/L, LDL = 1.9 mmol/L, triglycerides = 1.3 mmol/L, and HbA1C = 6.5% (48 mmol/mol).

Table 3.
Case # 3.

and uncontrollable bleeding from an open cut may not be suited to ingest black seed. Alternatively, the consumption of the black seed might exacerbate bleeding and could result in fatality. Consequently, the consumer may require hospitalization to receive additional medical care.

The majority of social media platforms consistently emphasize favorable testimonials from customers [81, 82]. Engaging in such a course of action will deceive the audience into believing that the product is both safe and cost-effective. Disseminating deceptive health information can inspire audiences to make erroneous decisions,

A male patient, 38 years old, complained of being unhealthy. The patient had been diagnosed with liver disorders and cardiovascular disease for the past 1 year. Due to that reason, he constantly consumed the following medications which were perindopril 4 mg, trimetazidine 35 mg, and glyceryl trinitrate 0.5 mg. In addition, he also consumed black seed, Annona muricata, omega 3, vitamin B complex (B1, B2, B3, B5, B6, B7, B9, and B12), and olive oil daily for 1 year. Laboratory tests performed before the consultation session showed the following abnormal readings, which were ESR =12, mean corpuscular hemoglobin (MCH) = 26, MCHC = 31, HbA1C = 6.1% (43 mmol/mol), total cholesterol = 6.1, LDL = 4.1 mmol/L, triglyceride = 2.1 mmol/L, AST = 44 U/L, ALT = 90 U/L, hs-C reactive protein (CRP) = 7.3 mg/L, LDH = 232, and rheumatoid factor (RF) = 15. The laboratory test showed that he might have liver disorders due to the consumption of black seed. For that reason, he was advised to discontinue the consumption of the black seed. It was recommended that he consume 200 mg of milk thistle twice daily for 6 months. Nonetheless, the post-laboratory test was not performed because the patient did not finish the milk thistle within the recommended time frame.

Table 4.
Case # 4

A 61-year-old male complained of chronic kidney disease. He was also diagnosed with diabetes mellitus Type 1 and cardiovascular disease. The patient had been prescribed the following medications: vildagliptin 50 mg, amlodipine 5 mg, bisoprolol 5 mg, calcium carbonate 500 mg, calcium polystyrene sulfonate powder, atorvastatin 40 mg, frusemide 40 mg, aspirin 100 mg, sodium bicarbonate powder, pantoprazole 40 mg and insulin Mixtard 30. In addition, he consumed black seed, olive oil, and kratom leaves for the past 3 years to eliminate signs and symptoms of hyperglycemia and cardiovascular disease. Laboratory tests obtained during the consultation session demonstrated the following abnormal readings: ESR = 75 mm/hr., red blood cell (RBC) = 3.3 X 10^{12}, Hb = 8.5 g/dL, PCV = 27, MCH = 26, RDW = 15.6, lymphocyte = 19%, FBS = 15 mmol/L, HbA1C = 7.9% (63 mmol/mol), urea = 21.3 mmol/L, creatinine = 401 umol/L, estimated glomerular filtration rate = 13 ml/min/1.73m^3, UA = 0.50 mmol/L, HDL = 0.91 mmol/L, CRP = 89.7 mg/L, ALP = 437 U/L, GGT = 176 iu/L, LDH = 321 U/L, protein urine trace = 2+, and glucose urine trace = 1+, positive blood in the urine. The results reflected that the patient potentially has liver disorders due to the black seed. For that reason, the patient was advised to consume 200 mg of milk thistle twice daily for 6 months and stop the consumption of black seed. The patient shall perform the following laboratory test after 6 months.

Table 5.
Case # 5.

resulting in detrimental health consequences such as false optimism, emotional turmoil, financial loss, and both internal and exterior physical injury [83]. The efficacy and safety of the product should be evaluated based on clinical data acquired from medical labs and medical assessments. Physicians should assume the responsibility of conducting the medical evaluation and determining if customers are free from medical conditions. Otherwise, the entrepreneurs would persist in disseminating health disinformation to the audiences, which would have detrimental effects on the healthcare system [84]. Furthermore, it is advisable for pharmacists to employ the STARZ-DRP technique to assess the drug-related requirements of consumers and detect any existing or possible drug-related issues among those who eat black seed [85–89]. Prior research has confirmed the effectiveness of this method in ensuring that pharmacists are able to carry out their responsibilities in a suitable way [90]. Pharmacists, acting as primary healthcare providers, can effectively avoid adverse consequences resulting from prolonged ingestion of black seed.

In short, doctors and pharmacists should resume the role of assessing, monitoring, and evaluating the consumption of health products. Physicians and pharmacists should have the knowledge and skills to report to the legal authorities about the findings of unwanted effects of black seed. Health misinformation poses a potential danger of exposing consumers to undesirable consequences. Consequently, it is imperative for the legal authorities to implement a regulation to prevent marketers from deceiving the public with false health information. Legal authorities have the authority to notify and prevent domestic marketers from promoting false or misleading health information on social media platforms.

5. Conclusion

Dissemination of inaccurate health information on social media has detrimental consequences for the healthcare system. Consumers may mistakenly see black seed as a safer and more cost-effective alternative to receiving professional treatment in a medical setting. They may believe that black seed has the potential to eradicate a diverse array of both minor and significant medical ailments. However, pursuing this line of action might potentially result in encountering additional detrimental consequences, ultimately leading to unnecessary hospital admissions and necessitating more comprehensive medical treatment. Consequently, this will lead customers to expend additional funds on a preventable medical condition. Hence, it is imperative for the legal authorities to oversee social media platforms in order to prevent the dissemination of health disinformation. Legal authorities should promote and advocate for consumers to obtain appropriate medical guidance prior to ingesting black seeds.

Conflict of interest

The author declares no conflict of interest.

Background of practice

The author utilizes an approach known as STARZ-DRP to assess, evaluate, and monitor patients' drug-related needs and drug-related problems.

Appreciation to my teammates who assisted in the completion of this article

1. Nur Aliah Binti Nazri, medical student at Kursk State of Medical University, Russian.

2. Nur Iman Binti Nazri, medical student at Kursk State of Medical University, Russian.

Author details

Nazri Nordin
Universiti Sains Malaysia, Malaysia

*Address all correspondence to: drnazrinordin@gmail.com;
dr.nazri.pharmacotherapeutic@gmail.com

IntechOpen

© 2024 The Author(s). Licensee IntechOpen. This chapter is distributed under the terms of the Creative Commons Attribution License (http://creativecommons.org/licenses/by/3.0), which permits unrestricted use, distribution, and reproduction in any medium, provided the original work is properly cited.

References

[1] Ventola CL. Social media and health care professionals: Benefits, risks, and best practices. P T. 2014;**39**(7):491-520

[2] Rajshri R, Malloy J. Evolving role of social Media in Health Promotion. In: Health Promotion—Principles and Approaches. London, UK: IntechOpen; 2023. DOI: 10.5772/intechopen.111967

[3] Abdelmoety ZH, Aboul-Dahab S, Agag G. A cross cultural investigation of retailers' commitment to CSR and customer citizenship behaviour: The role of ethical standard and value relevance. Journal of Retailing and Consumer Services. 2022;**64**:102796. DOI: 10.1016/j.jretconser.2021.102796

[4] Moorhead SA, Hazlet DE, Harrison L, et al. A new dimension of health care: Systemic review of the uses, benefits, and limitations of social media for health care professionals. Journal of Medical Internet Research. 2013;**15**(4):e85

[5] [Sunnah Barakah]. Herba Yang Diiktiraf Oleh World Health Organisation Sebagai Superfood [Video]. 2023. Available from: https://youtu.be/JeRmcpYdfmI?si=E-WTZZ7jSUlIYxHu

[6] [Adsolution]. Contoh Iklan Video Produk Kesihatan (Fizikal) [Video]. 2021. Available from: https://youtube.com/shorts/2-PExds6Fds?si=RV-aQVN9VYV0ee_r

[7] [dzulbahri]. E-Sacha Inchi Oil Dr Noordin Darus [Video]. 2022. Available from: https://youtube.com/shorts/_zQbJG5RJvI?si=4XR_kK69jyxup0Hc

[8] Vukušić Rukavina T, Viskić J, Machala Poplašen L, Relić D, Marelić M, Jokic D, et al. Dangers and benefits of social media on E-professionalism of health care professionals: Scoping review. Journal of Medical Internet Research. 2021;**23**(11):e25770. DOI: 10.2196/25770

[9] George DR. Making "social" safer: Are Facebook and other online networks becoming less hazardous for health professionals? The Journal of Clinical Ethics. 2012;**23**(4):348-352

[10] Suarez-Lledo V, Alvarez-Galvez J. Prevalence of health misinformation on social media: Systematic review. Journal of Medical Internet Research. 2021;**23**(1):e17187. DOI: 10.2196/17187

[11] Al-Balushi AA. In the era of social media: Is it time to establish a code of online ethical conduct for healthcare professionals? Sultan Qaboos University Medical Journal. 2020;**20**(1):e25-e28. DOI: 10.18295/squmj.2020.20.01.004. Epub 2020 Mar 9

[12] Yussof I, Ab Muin NF, Mohd M, Hatah E, Mohd Tahir NA, Mohamed SN. Breast cancer prevention and treatment misinformation on twitter: An analysis of two languages. Digital Health. 2023;**9**:20552076231205742. DOI: 10.1177/20552076231205742

[13] Mohamad E, Tham JS, Mohd Ajis SZ, Hamzah MR, Ayub SH, Tri Sakti AM, et al. Exposure to misinformation, risk perception, and confidence towards the government as factors influencing negative attitudes towards COVID-19 vaccination in Malaysia. International Journal of Environmental Research and Public Health. 2022;**19**(22):14623. DOI: 10.3390/ijerph192214623

[14] Balakrishnan V, Ng WZ, Soo MC, Han GJ, Lee CJ. Infodemic and fake news—A comprehensive overview of its global magnitude during the

COVID-19 pandemic in 2021: A scoping review. International Journal of Disaster Risk Reduction. 2022;**78**:103144. DOI: 10.1016/j.ijdrr.2022.103144. Epub 2022 Jul 1

[15] Shroff SM, Sreeramareddy CT. Marketing claims, promotional strategies, and product information on Malaysian e-cigarette retailer websites-a content analysis. Substance Abuse Treatment, Prevention, and Policy. 2024;**19**:11. DOI: 10.1186/s13011-024-00592-z

[16] Wahab MSA, Hamdi H, Ali AA, Karuppannan M, Zulkifli MH, Maniam S, et al. The use of herbal and dietary supplements for COVID-19 prevention: A survey among the public in a Malaysian suburban town. Journal of Herbal Medicine. 2023;**39**:100650. DOI: 10.1016/j.hermed.2023.100650. Epub 2023 Mar 22

[17] Martinez LS, Hughes S, Walsh-Buhi ER, Tsou M. "Okay, we get it. You vape": An analysis of geocoded content, context, and sentiment regarding E-cigarettes on Twitter. Journal of Health Communication. 2018;**23**(6):550-562. DOI: 10.1080/10810730.2018.1493057

[18] Merianos AL, Gittens OE, Mahabee-Gittens EM. Depiction of health effects of electronic cigarettes on YouTube. Journal of Substance Use. 2016;**21**(6):614-619. DOI: 10.3109/14659891.2015.1118565

[19] Laestadius LI, Wahl MM, Cho YI. #Vapelife: An exploratory study of electronic cigarette use and promotion on Instagram. Substance Use & Misuse. 2016;**51**(12):1669-1673. DOI: 10.1080/10826084.2016.1188958

[20] Keim-Malpass J, Mitchell EM, Sun E, Kennedy C. Using twitter to understand public perceptions regarding the #HPV vaccine: Opportunities for public health nurses to engage in social marketing. Public Health Nursing. 2017;**34**(4):316-323. DOI: 10.1111/phn.12318

[21] Guidry JPD, Carlyle K, Messner M, Jin Y. On pins and needles: How vaccines are portrayed on Pinterest. Vaccine. 2015;**33**(39):5051-5056. DOI: 10.1016/j.vaccine.2015.08.064

[22] Becker BFH, Larson HJ, Bonhoeffer J, van Mulligen EM, Kors JA, Sturkenboom MCJM. Evaluation of a multinational, multilingual vaccine debate on twitter. Vaccine. 2016;**34**(50):6166-6171. DOI: 10.1016/j.vaccine.2016.11.007

[23] Bora K, Das D, Barman B, Borah P. Are internet videos useful sources of information during global public health emergencies? A case study of YouTube videos during the 2015-16 Zika virus pandemic. Pathogens and Global Health. 2018;**112**(6):320-328. DOI: 10.1080/20477724.2018.1507784

[24] Guidry JP, Jin Y, Orr CA, Messner M, Meganck S. Ebola on Instagram and twitter: How health organizations address the health crisis in their social media engagement. Public Relations Review. 2017;**43**(3):477-486. DOI: 10.1016/j.pubrev.2017.04.009

[25] Morin C, Bost I, Mercier A, Dozon J, Atlani-Duault L. Information circulation in times of Ebola: Twitter and the sexual transmission of Ebola by survivors. PLoS Currents. 2018;**10**. DOI: 10.1371/currents.outbreaks.4e35a9446b89c1b46f8308099840d48f

[26] Menon D, Chelakkot PG, Sunil D, Lakshmaiah A. A cross sectional review of patient information available in the world wide web on CyberKnife: Fallacies and pitfalls. Supportive Care in Cancer. 2017;**25**(12):3769-3773. DOI: 10.1007/s00520-017-3807-4

[27] Abukaraky A, Hamdan A, Ameera M, Nasief M, Hassona Y. Quality of YouTube TM videos on dental implants. Medicina Oral, Patología Oral y Cirugía Bucal. 2018;**23**(4):e463-e468. DOI: 10.4317/medoral.22447

[28] Vosoughi S, Roy D, Aral S. The spread of true and false news online. Science. 2018;**359**(6380):1146-1151. DOI: 10.1126/science.aap9559

[29] Levy J, Strombeck R. Health benefits and risks of the internet. Journal of Medical Systems. 2002;**26**(6):495-510. DOI: 10.1023/a:1020288508362

[30] Pharmaceutical Services, Ministry of Health Malaysia. How to Identify Medicines That Are Registered with MOH? Available from: https://pharmacy.moh.gov.my/en/faq/how-identify-medicines-are-registered-moh.html [Accessed: February, 2024].

[31] National Pharmaceutical Regulatory Agency, Ministry of Health Malaysia. Roles and Functions. Available from: https://www.npra.gov.my/index.php/en/ [Accessed: February, 2024]

[32] National Pharmaceutical Regulatory Agency, Ministry of Health Malaysia. Guideline on Natural Products and Therapeutic Claim. Available from: https://www.npra.gov.my/index.php/en/guidelines-for-natural-products/1527280-drgd-appendix-7b-guideline-on-natural-products-with-therapeutic-claim.html [Accessed: February, 2024]

[33] National Pharmaceutical Regulatory Agency, Ministry of Health Malaysia. Guideline on Registration of Health Supplements. Available from: https://www.npra.gov.my/images/00NPRA/health-supplements/appendix4HS.pdf [Accessed: February, 2024]

[34] National Pharmaceutical Regulatory Agency, Ministry of Health Malaysia. Report on Suspected Adverse Drug Reactions. Available from: https://www.npra.gov.my/easyarticles/images/users/1066/ADR%20Reporting/ADR_Form_Healthcare_Prof_web.pdf [Accessed: February, 2024]

[35] Ahmad A, Husain A, Mujeeb M, Khan SA, Najmi AK, Siddique NA, et al. A review on therapeutic potential of *Nigella sativa*: A miracle herb. Asian Pacific Journal of Tropical Biomedicine. 2013;**3**(5):337-352. DOI: 10.1016/S2221-1691(13)60075-1

[36] Ziaee T, Moharreri N, Hosseinzadeh H. Review of pharmacological and toxicological effects of *Nigella sativa* and its active constituents. The Journal of Medicinal Plants Studies. 2012;**2**(42):16-42

[37] Shafiq H, Ahmad A, Masud T, Kaleem M. Cardio-protective and anti-cancer therapeutic potential of *Nigella sativa*. Iranian Journal of Basic Medical Sciences. 2014;**17**(12):967-979

[38] Butt MS, Sultan MT. *Nigella sativa*: Reduces the risk of various maladies. Critical Reviews in Food Science and Nutrition. 2010;**50**(7):654-665. DOI: 10.1080/10408390902768797

[39] Ali Salim LZ, Othman R, Abdulla MA, et al. Thymoquinone inhibits murine leukemia WEHI-3 cells in vivo and in vitro. PLoS One. 2014;**9**(12):e115340

[40] Khader M, Bresgen N, Eckl PM. In vitro toxicological properties of thymoquinone. Food and Chemical Toxicology. 2009;**47**(1):129-133

[41] Pathan SA, Jain GK, Zaidi SMA, et al. Stability-indicating ultra-performance liquid chromatography method for the estimation of thymoquinone and its application in biopharmaceutical studies. Biomedical Chromatography. 2011;**25**(5):613-620

[42] Ibraheim ZZ. Effect of *Nigella sativa* seeds and total oil on some blood parameters in female volunteers. Saudi Pharmaceutical Journal. 2002;**10**:54-59

[43] Ahmad B, Masud T, Uppal AM, Naveed AK. Effects of *Nigella sativa* oil on some blood parameters in type 2 diabetes mellitus patients. Asian Journal of Chemistry. 2009;**21**:5373-5381

[44] Alsamarai A, Abdulsatar M, Alobaidi A. Evaluation of topical black seed oil in the treatment of allergic rhinitis. Antiinflammatory Antiallergy Agents in Medicinal Chemistry. 2014;**13**:75-82. DOI: 10.2174/18715230113129990014

[45] Bamosa AO, Kaatabi H, Lebda FM, Al Elq AM, Al-Sultan A. Effect of *Nigella sativa* seeds on the glycemic control of patients with type 2 diabetes mellitus. Indian Journal of Physiology and Pharmacology. 2010;**54**:344-354

[46] Kaplan SA, Meehan AG, Shah A. The age related decrease in testosterone is significantly exacerbated in obese men with the metabolic syndrome. What are the implications for the relatively high incidence of erectile dysfunction observed in these men? The Journal of Urology. 2006;**176**:1524-1528. DOI: 10.1016/j.juro.2006.06.003

[47] Fallah HH, Amini M, Mohtashami R, Ghamarchehre ME, Sadeqhi Z, Kianbakht S, et al. Blood pressure lowering effect of *Nigella sativa* l. seed oil in healthy volunteers: A randomized, double-blind, placebo-controlled clinical trial. Phytotherapy Research. 2013;**27**:1849-1853. DOI: 10.1002/ptr.4944

[48] Dehkordi FR, Kamkhah AF. Antihypertensive effect of *Nigella sativa* seed extract in patients with mild hypertension. Fundamental & Clinical Pharmacology. 2008;**22**:447-452. DOI: 10.1111/j.1472-8206.2008.00607.x

[49] Yimer EM, Tuem KB, Karim A, Ur-Rehman N, Anwar F, Nigella sativa L. (black cumin): A promising natural remedy for wide range of illnesses. Evidence-Based Complementary and Alternative Medicine. 2019;**2019**:1528635. DOI: 10.1155/2019/1528635

[50] Ong YS, Saiful Yazan L, Ng WK, Noordin MM, Sapuan S, Foo JB, et al. Acute and subacute toxicity profiles of thymoquinone-loaded nanostructured lipid carrier in BALB/c mice. International Journal of Nanomedicine. 2016;**11**:5905-5915. DOI: 10.2147/IJN.S114205

[51] Ali B, Amin S, Ahmad J, Ali A, Ali M, Mir SR. Bioavailability enhancement studies of amoxicillin with Nigella. The Indian Journal of Medical Research. 2012;**135**:555-559

[52] Al-Jenoobi FI, Al-Thukair AA, Alam MA, Abbas FA, Al-Mohizea AM, Alkharfy KM, et al. Effect of curcuma longa on CYP2D6- and CYP3A4-mediated metabolism of dextromethorphan in human liver Microsomes and healthy human subjects. European Journal of Drug Metabolism and Pharmacokinetics. 2015;**40**:61-66. DOI: 10.1007/s13318-014-0180-2

[53] Al-Ali A, Alkhawajah AA, Randhawa MA, Shaikh NA. Oral and intraperitoneal LD50 of thymoquinone, an active principle of *Nigella sativa*, in mice and rats. Journal of Ayub Medical College, Abbottabad. 2008;**20**:25-27

[54] Nagi MN, Almakki HA. Thymoquinone supplementation induces quinone reductase and glutathione transferase in mice liver: Possible role in protection against chemical carcinogenesis and toxicity. Phytotherapy Research. 2009;**23**(9):1295-1298

[55] Pottoo FH, Ibrahim AM, Alammar A, Alsinan R, Aleid M, Alshehhi A, et al.

Thymoquinone: Review of its potential in the treatment of neurological diseases. Pharmaceuticals. 2022;**15**(4):408. DOI: 10.3390/ph15040408

[56] Alkharfy KM, Ahmad A, Khan RM, Al-Shagha WM. Pharmacokinetic plasma behaviors of intravenous and oral bioavailability of thymoquinone in a rabbit model. European Journal of Drug Metabolism and Pharmacokinetics. 2015;**40**(3):319-323

[57] Arslan E, Sayin S, Demirbas S, Cakar M, Somak NG, Yesilkaya S, et al. A case study report of acute renal failure associated with *Nigella sativa* in a diabetic patient. Journal of Integrative Medicine. 2013;**11**(1):64-66. DOI: 10.3736/jintegrmed2013010

[58] [flavours.oflifewtihsasha]. 9 benefits of blackseeds (kalonji) [Video]. 2022. Available from: https://youtube.com/shorts/2ucJTXxF14Q?si=EGnlUV1mMuGy3_w6

[59] [MantaBSMI Health]. Habbatussauda/Jintan Hitam—Manfaat & Dosisnya untuk Kesehatan [Video]. 2019. Available from: https://youtu.be/W2n3p0NIeeM?si=2YyvNTUZbv1Zm3U9

[60] [Dr Noordin Darus]. 17 Manfaat dan Rahsia Habbatul Sauda! [Video]. 2021. Available from: https://youtu.be/69QEhXsGE-I?si=lki_ra6UvRSQF3Iz

[61] [dr.Emas uperr]. Health Benefits and Dangers of Habbatussauda/Black Cumin [Video]. 2024. Available from: https://youtu.be/mkaR7Y2DJHk?si=GwOfRc4uXd5e0i7v

[62] [Dokter Fery TV]. Habbatussauda (Jintan Hitam) Mempunyai Manfaat Yang Baik Untuk Kesehatan [Video]. 2023. Available from: https://youtu.be/oycuCbCf7mc?si=sWv5UivEOUyba99A

[63] [dr. Zaidul Akbar Official]. Dahsyatnya Habatusaudah & Bakteri [Video]. 2023. Available from: https://youtu.be/T742170mNkk?si=-7l9GXvYmLmFQsxJ

[64] [Sumardi Sahari Official]. Ketahui Manfaat Potensial dan Efek Samping dari Habbatussauda [Video]. 2022. Available from: https://youtu.be/AIHCsdd20zo?si=YpdllNpbj5WdCrmu

[65] [Khalid Basalamah Official]. Thibbun Nabawi—Habbatussaudah (Jintan Hitam) [Video]. 2022. Available from: https://youtu.be/cH600GIwBA8?si=L-31Llx7h2vX6F_w

[66] [Aiwah HQ]. Habbatussauda: Dari cepat penat, lesu, sakit sendi & fibroid. Kini semuanya kembali sembuh! [Video]. 2023. Available from: https://youtu.be/OVWPuY4p6M0?si=-PM05QBEIqmOHUB7

[67] [CNN Indonesia]. Ragam Manfaat Habbatussauda [Video]. 2020. Available from: https://youtu.be/QOOkWQ2Zu7U?si=1lZX73vkg6mZ3fhz

[68] Heineman B, Jewell M, Moran M, Bradley K, Spitzer KA, Lindenauer PK. Content analysis of promotional material for asthma-related products and therapies on Instagram. Allergy, Asthma and Clinical Immunology. 2021;**17**(1):26. DOI: 10.1186/s13223-021-00528-3

[69] [Pharmaceutical Services Ministry of Health Malaysia]. Penalty. Available from: https://pharmacy.moh.gov.my/ms/entri/hukuman.html [Accessed: March 13, 2024]

[70] [Poison Act 1952]. ACT 290 Medicines (Advertisement and Sale) Act 1956 (Revised—1983). Available from: https://pharmacy.moh.gov.my/sites/default/files/document-upload/medicine-advertisement-sale-act-1956-

act-290_3.pdf [Accessed: March 13, 2024]

[71] [motivationaldoc]. 30 Miracle Healing Benefits of Black Seed Oil—Dr. Alan Mandell, D.C. [Video]. 2017. Available from: https://youtu.be/9Aop5fq4qsk, "30 Miracle Healing Benefits of Black Seed Oil"

[72] [Ryan Taylor]. 10 Amazing Benefits of Black Seed Oil [Video]. 2023. Available from: https://youtu.be/EgnaWFN4XhM?si=-g6ku_r2QqXvpz2J

[73] [Healthy Sloth]. Black Cumin Seed Oil Benefits—Kalonji Oil Benefits and Health use [Video]. 2019. Available from: https://youtu.be/hkz-BkKrjW0?si=_PkaoMILgDKuedt8

[74] [HALAL2U Marketing]. Minyak Habbatus Sauda Ekstrak Fraksi Kaya. 2021. Available from: https://www.sawdapremium.com/?gad_source=1&gclid=Cj0KCQjwncWvBhD_ARIsAEb2HW8tc8nWpwW6krkZ-afEAHDyc8N1Po0Nkh8_3BiXxbzkxpH1LRicmg0aAk6QEALw_wcB [Accessed: March 14, 2024]

[75] [Galeri Addeen]. Habbatus Sauda Sahara Black Seed Turkey. 2024. Available from: https://galeriaddeen.com/product/habbatus-sauda-sahara-black-seed-turkey/ [Accessed: March 14, 2024]

[76] [Aafiyat]. Info Aafiyat: Kajian Menarik Berkaitan Minyak Habbatus Sauda & Masalah Buah Pinggang. 2021. Available from: https://search.aafiyatgroup.com/view/8a3g5GE1V0yPpGlDeP/info-aafiyat-kajian-menarik-berkaitan-minyak-habbatus-sauda-masalah-buah-pinggang?q=&type= [Accessed: March 14, 2024]

[77] Hamdan A, Haji Idrus R, Mokhtar MH. Effects of *Nigella Sativa* on Type-2 diabetes mellitus: A systematic review. International Journal of Environmental Research and Public Health. 2019;**16**(24):4911. DOI: 10.3390/ijerph16244911

[78] Wang X, Jiang A, Batra V. Severe thrombocytopenia associated with black seed oil and evening primrose oil. Cureus. 2020;**12**(6):e8390. DOI: 10.7759/cureus.8390

[79] Maideen NMP, Balasubramanian R, Ramanathan S. *Nigella Sativa* (black seeds), a potential herb for the pharmacotherapeutic management of hypertension—A review. Current Cardiology Reviews. 2021;**17**(4):e230421187786. DOI: 10.2174/1573403X16666201110125906

[80] Khan MA, Chen HC, Tania M, Zhang DZ. Anticancer activities of *Nigella sativa* (black cumin). African Journal of Traditional, Complementary, and Alternative Medicines. 2011;**8**(5 Suppl):226-232. DOI: 10.4314/ajtcam.v8i5S.10 Epub 2011 Jul 3

[81] [Habatussauda_Noraslina]. Habbatussauda sangat mujarab untuk meningkatkan system pertahanan dan Kesihatan badan [Facebook]. 2022. Available from: https://web.facebook.com/watch/?v=726415608321720 [Accessed: March 15, 2024]

[82] Testimoni Habbatus-Sauda [Facebook]. 2014. Available from: https://web.facebook.com/barakahfood/posts/testimoni-habbatus-sauda1-pn-fatimah-pembuangan-air-besar-lawas-keluar-lemak-lem/614937738623922/?_rdc=1&_rdr [Accessed: March 15, 2024]

[83] Fridman I, Johnson S, Elston LJ. Health information and misinformation: A framework to guide research and practice. JMIR Medical Education. 2023;**9**:e38687. DOI: 10.2196/38687

[84] Sylvia Chou WY, Gaysynsky A, Cappella JN. Where we go from here: Health misinformation on social media. American Journal of Public Health. 2020;**110**(S3):S273-S275. DOI: 10.2105/AJPH.2020.305905

[85] Sarriff A, Nordin N, Hassali MA. STARZ-DRP: A step-by-step approach for pharmacy triage services. Malaysian Journal of Pharmacy. 2011;**1**(9):311-326

[86] Nordin N, Sarriff A, Hassali MA. STARZ-DRP: A tool for pharmacy triage services. Asian Journal of Pharmaceutical and Clinical Research. 2017;**10**(10):151-157

[87] Nordin N, Hassali MA, Sarriff A. STARZ-DRP: A structured framework for teaching community pharmacists to counsel self-care customers. International Journal of Pharmacy and Pharmaceutical Sciences. 2017;**9**(12):271-275

[88] Sarriff A, Hassali MA, Nordin N. Introduction to 'STARZ-DRP': A Step-by-Step Approach for Triaging Decision in Community Pharmacy. School of Pharmaceutical Sciences, Universiti Sains Malaysia; 2015. p. 15. ISBN: 978-967-13162-2-1

[89] Nordin N, Hassali MA. STARZ-DRP: Improving Efficiency of Patient Care in Community Pharmacies. London, UK: InTechOpen; 2020. DOI: 10.5772/intechopen.86021

[90] Nazri N, Mohamed Azmi H, Azmi S. STARZ-DRP: A Community Pharmacist Approach as a Medication Protector. Universiti Sains Malaysia; 2021. pp. 66-68. e-ISBN 978-967-461-639-7